Fitness Manual for Women Over 50

A Guide for Women to Always Stay Active and Make the Weight Loss possible by adopting Healthy Lifestyle Habits, Soft Training, and Best Fitness Exercises

By

Dylan Bold

Thanks for choosing this book. Your opinion on this manuscript will always be welcome. You will enrich my work, and I will appreciate your kindness. Enjoy the reading!

https://www.amazon.com/review/create-review/ref=cm_cr_othr_d_wr_but_top?ie=UTF8&channel=glance-detail&asin=B086BNV752

Table Of Contents

Introduction

Physical fitness is the state of health and well-being and, more precisely, the ability to perform the sport, profession, and day-to-day activities aspects. In general, physical fitness is accomplished by proper nutrition, moderate-vigorous physical exercise, and enough rest. Physical fitness has been shown to have positive effects on the blood pressure of the body because staying active and exercising regularly creates a stronger heart. Physical activity strengthens the immune system. Physical activity can boost fitness and mental health. It would help if you stayed active as you get older. Regular physical activity could help you stay healthy and strong. For older women, physical activity provides many advantages. Many women of all ages, sizes, and abilities should get moderate-intensity aerobic physical activity at least 2 hours and 30 minutes each week. It would help if you also had exercises that improve your muscle on at least two days each week.

For all women, balancing exercises are necessary, but particularly of older women at higher risk of falls. In older women, weight lifting can be the best way to maintain overall fitness and avoid the slow creeping rise in fat.

Keeping fit is important at any age, but exercising more than 50 years is important for maintaining a healthy lifestyle as you age. There's no justification that at 50, you can't look as fit and beautiful as at 40, but there's one hitch: once they reach this landmark era, even stars with personal trainers and diet coaches have to work a bit harder to lose the pounds. You'll have to put extra effort into one of the main reasons: your body composition changes as you age.

Every ten years after age 35, you lose muscle mass at an average rate of 3-5 percent, and this can affect the way you burn fat. "The body is going through aging as it leaves the rising one." The body doesn't need as much energy as it used to when this happens. What's more, they take their toll all those years of playing sports, chasing after your kids, and walking up and down stairways. You can note that your joints are a little stiffer than they were a few decades ago, and your muscles are a little more sorry. Then, there's your ever-evolving metabolism problem.

You are resting on the metabolic rate, the capacity of your body to burn fat sitting on the sofa doing nothing decreases by around 1-2 percent per decade due to loss of muscle mass and increased fat mass.

Generally, our diets don't change enough to compensate for this metabolic transition, ensuring that with every birthday weight will slowly but surely creep up. "There are a variety of roadblocks that people will face while trying to lose weight in their 50s," "But once you know what they are— and how to get around them— it's easy to succeed in falling pounds." One of the good things you can do at any age is to change your routine and try something new. Even if in your life you've never picked up a dumbbell, now's the best time to learn how to use the weight room (but please, if you're a newbie, first work with a trainer, so you don't injure yourself!).

Because the trick to losing weight over 50 is this: Create more muscle mass to improve your metabolism (you now have about 20 percent less than when you were 20). "The good news is that with a well-structured weight-training routine, you can turn all of this around." That will help you recover the capacity to lose weight just as you did 20 years ago.

Get weights lifted at least twice a week, whether you are using free weights or equipment or doing bodyweight exercises. Lifting every day doesn't hurt — make sure you work for different muscle groups or exercise each day differently.

The nutrition of a person after 50 is crucial. It is the most important factor, undoubtedly, in maintaining a healthy body at this age. In the form of junk food, inactivity, and too much alcohol, it cannot tolerate far more violence. The side effects are expected. Good nutrition is important throughout the entire lifespan, of course. Still, around and after age 50, changes take place inside the body that makes the food you eat of particular significance, "As you age, you lose muscle mass, around 10 percent every decade after age 50." "When you lose your muscle, you are more likely to gain body fat and needless calories," she says, "because the muscle consumes more calories than body fat. Prioritizing exercise is also important — especially resistance training to help counteract the decline in metabolism that happens with aging. Nutrition must be given priority to avoid heart disease, diabetes, and other diseases that are of greater concern as people grow older.

When women approach 50, their bodies plan for menopause and go through other side effects of aging. Most people need to follow new and different strategies to preserve their health, including changing their diets to get the nutrients they need. We may want to look at the best diets for women over 50, in that case. The 50s, due to pre-menopause and menopause, are a time for big changes.

This is a time in a woman's life in which she has hormone variations, which can cause metabolism and body weight changes.

Kay also discusses osteoporosis, osteoarthritis, and changes in the regulation of blood sugar (insulin resistance may occur due to changes in hormones), as other disorders women may experience in this age group. Losing weight after being 50 years old is no easy feat. At the end of a hard day, not only are sugar treats enticing, but your metabolism has probably taken a nose-dive too. From the age of 20, the metabolism is slowing by about 2 percent every decade. You can understand why by the time you reach middle age, the scale is creeping up more easily. Yet all hope is not lost. Many ways to boost your metabolism easily, including the easiest approach you can start today. After 50, if you were physically active, this is perfect. But if you haven't regularly exercised, it's not too late to start.

Physical activity can help to alleviate some of the menopause symptoms— hot flashes, joint pain, and sleep problems. Exercise reduces the risk of cardiac disease and osteoporosis. Additionally, it helps to control weight and absorbs fat in the belly. The effects of exercise are so strong that each physiological function in the body is affected for the better.

For those of you who have purchased the audiobook, you may ask for a pdf for references of exercises described later in the book, by sending an email to "dylan.bold.author@gmail.com".

Chapter 1: Introduction to Physical Fitness

1.1 What is Physical Fitness?

Physical fitness is the state of health and well-being and, more precisely, the ability to perform a sport, profession, and day-to-day activities aspects. In general, physical fitness is achieved through proper nutrition, moderate-vigorous physical exercise, and enough rest. Before the industrial revolution, fitness was described as the capacity without excessive fatigue to carry out the activities of the day. With automation and improvements in lifestyles, however, physical fitness is now considered a measure of the Body's ability to act effectively and efficiently in work and leisure activities, to be safe, to tolerate hypokinetic diseases, and to respond to emergencies. Fitness is defined as the fitness standard or state. About 1950, perhaps by the Industrial Revolution and World War II treatise, the word "fitness" increased by a factor of ten in the western vernacular.

The modern fitness definition describes either the ability of a person or machine to perform a specific function or a holistic human adaptability definition to deal with different situations. This has led to social fitness and attractiveness interrelationship that mobilized the global fitness and fitness equipment industries. Fitness is applied to individuals with substantial aerobic or anaerobic capacity, i.e., endurance or strength, concerning a specific function.

A well-rounded fitness program enhances a person in all aspects of fitness compared to only one practice, such as cardiorespiratory endurance or weight training alone. A structured individual-specific fitness program usually focuses on one or more focused abilities, and age-or health-related needs, such as bone health.

Many outlets also cite mental, social, and emotional wellbeing as an integral part of overall fitness. For textbooks, this is often described as a three-point triangle reflecting physical, social, and mental health. Physical fitness can also avoid or cure several chronic health conditions induced by an unhealthy lifestyle or aging. Working out can also help some people to sleep better and can potentially relieve some mood disorders in some people. Developing work has shown that many of the exercise's benefits are transmitted through the role of the skeletal muscle as an endocrine organ. That is, contracting muscles release several substances known as myokines, facilitating the growth of new tissue, tissue repair, and other anti-inflammatory functions, which in effect reduce the risk of developing different inflammatory conditions.

Adults should engage in moderate-intensity at least 150 minutes a week, or 75 minutes a week of moderate aerobic physical activity, or an equivalent combination of moderate and vigorous-intensity aerobic activity for significant health benefits. Aerobic exercise should be done in episodes of at least 10 minutes, and should ideally be distributed over the week. The level we exercise at is essential, and light activity such as strolling and housework It unlikely to have a positive impact substantially on most people's health. To be useful for aerobic exercise, it must elevate heart rate and induce suddenness. Everyone should do a moderate-intensity aerobic exercise for at least 150 minutes a week, but that is only the minimum for health benefits. If you do that more than 150 minutes, you'll reap even more health benefits. Sedentary time is terrible for the health of everyone, and no amount of exercise will counteract the effects of sitting for too long. Such standards now align even better than those used in the US, which also covers muscle-building and bone-strengthening exercises such as lifting weights and yoga tips.

Adults should increase their aerobic activity to 300 minutes (5 hours) a moderate-intensity week, or 160 minutes in a week of vigorous-intensity aerobic exercise, or an equivalent combination of moderate and vigorous-intensity Additional and broader wellbeing benefits. Beyond this number, other health benefits are obtained by participating in physical activity. Adults should also do moderate or high-intensity muscle-strengthening activities. This includes all major muscle groups on two or three days a week as additional health benefits are given by these activities. Physical fitness consists of 11 parts-6 of them related to health and five related to ability. All the pieces, including sports, are essential to excellent performance in physical activity. But the six are named contributing to health-related physical fitness because kinesiology scientists have shown that they can reduce your risk of chronic illness and promote good health and wellness. Such components of fitness are a composition of the body, cardiorespiratory endurance, flexibility, muscle endurance, power, and energy. Also, they help you to function effectively in everyday activities. As the name implies, skill-related components of physical fitness enable you to perform well in sports and other activities that require motor skills. For starters, speed helps you in such sports as track and field. Such five elements of physical fitness are also correlated with health but less so than the components related to health. Of example, balance, endurance, and coordination in older adults are essential in avoiding falls (a primary health concern), and reaction time are correlated with the risk of automobile accidents. The following two features describe each part of physical fitness in more detail: This includes all major muscle groups on two or three days a week as additional health benefits are given by these activities.

Think about a runner. Perhaps she can run a long distance without tiring; thus, she has practical fitness in at least one field of physical fitness related to health. But is she getting good fitness in all six parts? Running is an outstanding form of physical activity, but becoming a runner does not guarantee success in all areas of physical exercise-related to safety. As the runner, you may be more fit in some parts of fitness than in others. Much as the runner in our example does not receive a high rating in all parts of physical fitness related to health, she may not score the same for all parts of physical fitness related to ability. While most sports require several skill-related parts of fitness, different games may require different parts. A skater can have outstanding endurance, for example, but lack adequate reaction speed. In some cases, some people have more natural abilities than in others. You should enjoy any type of physical activity, no matter how you perform on the skill-related parts of physical fitness. Do note that good health in skill-related physical exercise doesn't come from being perfect. It comes from doing workouts designed to improve physical fitness related to your health, and it can be experienced by great athletes as well as by people who consider themselves bad athletes. As noted earlier, exercise linked to health provides a twofold benefit. Not only does it help you to remain healthy, but it also helps you to do well in sports and other activities. Cardiorespiratory fitness, for example, helps you overcome heart failure and lets you do well in activities such as swimming and cross-country running. Similarly, strength allows you to perform well in sports like football and wrestling, muscle endurance is critical in soccer and tennis, flexibility helps in sports like gymnastics and diving, power helps in track activities like discus throwing and long jumping, and having a healthy amount of body fat makes the body more effective in many activities. All women have essential physical activity during their lives. Read on how you can adjust your routine of physical activity to suit your needs depending on your age, stage of life, or physical ability. If you are overweight and want to begin a workout, start moving around your home slowly. Seek stretching or weight lifting while watching TV. You can lift food canisters, water jugs, or other household objects as weights. Walking in a safe area near where you stay is a perfect way to start doing more exercise for women of all ages or types. You don't need special athletic equipment or accessories, only comfortable walking shoes. Start at least three days a week with 1 minute walks at a comfortable pace. Add more walking minutes and increasing how quickly you walk as your body becomes accustomed to the practice.

1.2 Why is Fitness Important for Women?

You must stay active as you get older. Regular physical activity might help you stay healthy and strong. For older women, physical exercise offers many advantages.

- Preventing bone loss and muscle
- Reducing the risk of breaking bones,
- Helping avoid or postpone conditions such as diabetes and cardiac disease,
- Reducing joint swelling and arthritis pain,
- Reducing anxiety and depression symptoms
- Helping you stay independent for longer,

Women of all ages, sizes, and abilities should get moderate-intensity aerobic physical activity at least 2 hours and 30 minutes each week. You also need exercises that improve your muscle on at least two days each week. For all women, balancing exercises are necessary, but particularly of older women at higher risk of falls. It includes women who have fallen or have trouble walking in the recent past. Doing balance and muscle-strengthening exercises for at least 1 hour and 30 minutes a week helps to fewer the risk of falling and getting injured.

Examples of such activities include tai chi, backward walking, and standing from a sitting position. Getting active will help you live a happier, longer life. Learn exercises and stretches to improve your health at any age.

Controlling Blood Pressure

Physical fitness has been shown to have positive effects on the blood pressure of the body because staying active and exercising produces a healthier heart regularly. The heart is the main organ responsible for systolic blood pressure and diastolic blood pressure. Getting involved in physical activity increases blood pressure. Once the operation is halted, blood pressure returns to normal. The more physical activity one participates in, the simpler this cycle becomes, resulting in the person being more' fit.' The heart does not work as hard through regular physical exercise to produce an increase in blood pressure that reduces the strain on the arteries and decreases the overall blood pressure.

Cancer Prevention

Disease control and prevention centers provide lifestyle guidelines for maintaining a balanced diet and engaging in physical activity to reduce disease risk. Be as lean as possible, and do not get underweight. Adults will participate in at least 150 minutes of moderate physical activity or 75 minutes of intense physical activity each week. Children will engage in moderate or severe physical activity for at least one hour every week. Be involved physically every day, for at least thirty minutes. Evite sugar, and limit energy-packed food consumption.

Control your diet with a variety of vegetables, grains, fruits, legumes, etc.

Restrict sodium intake, Red meat consumption, and processed meat consumption. Limit alcoholic drinks for men to two, and women to one per day.

Daily physical activity is a factor that helps reduce blood pressure in a person and increases the levels of cholesterol, two key components that correlate with heart disease and type 2 diabetes. Furthermore, because it is a multifactorial disease, physical fitness is a controllable treatment, it is known cancer is not a disease and can only be cured by physical exercise; the broad correlations linked to being physically fit and lowering the risk of cancer are enough to provide a strategy to reduce the risk of cancer. Such classifications of physical activity take into account the deliberate workout, and essential tasks are conducted daily to give the public a greater understanding of what fitness levels are sufficient to prevent potential diseases.

Inflammation

The result of increased physical activity and decreased inflammation. It induces an inflammatory response in the short term and an anti-inflammatory reaction in the long term. Physical activity, in conjunction with or regardless of changes in body weight, reduces inflammation. The mechanisms which link physical activity to inflammation, however, are unknown.

Immune System

Physical activity strengthens the immune system. It depends on the concentration of endogenous factors (such as sex hormones, metabolic hormones, and growth hormones), body temperature, blood flow, and body position, and hydration status. Physical activity has shown that natural killer (NK) cells, NK T cells, macrophages, neutrophils, and eosinophil's, supplements, cytokines, antibodies, and T cytotoxic cells have increased levels. The mechanism which links physical activity to the immune system is not fully understood, though.

Weight Control

Resilience by physical fitness facilitates a vast and complex variety of health benefits. Individuals who maintain physical fitness standards typically control their body fat distribution and stay away from obesity. The abdominal fat, especially visceral fat, is most directly affected by aerobic exercise. Strength training has been known to increase muscle levels in the body, but it can also reduce body fat. Factors that mediate metabolism in relation to abdominal fat are sex steroid hormones, insulin, and adequate immune response. Physical fitness thus provides weight control by controlling certain body functions.

Menopause and Physical Fitness

Menopause is often said to have happened when a woman has not had vaginal bleeding from her last menstrual cycle for more than a year. There are a variety of menopause-related symptoms, most of which affect a woman's quality of life involved in this stage of her life. Exercising is one way to reduce the severity of the symptoms and maintain a healthy fitness level. There may be physical, hormonal, or internal changes to the body before and during menopause as the female body shifts. With regular exercise, those improvements can be minimized or even stopped. Such modifications include:

Preventing weight gain: Women around menopause tend to experience a decrease in muscle mass and an increase in fat. Increasing the amount of physical exercise done can help prevent such changes.

Reducing the risk of developing breast cancer: Weight loss resulting from regular exercise can protect against breast cancer.

Strengthening bones: Physical activity may slow menopause-related bone loss, decreasing the chance of osteoporosis and bone fractures.

Reducing the risk of disease: More weight can increase the risk of heart disease and type 2 diabetes and may be offset by regular physical activity

Boosting mood. Women who reported being physically active at the beginning each day were 49 percent less likely to have experienced uncomfortable hot flushes. This is in contrast to women whose activity levels declined and were more likely to experience uncomfortable hot flushes.

Mental Health

Physical activity can boost fitness and mental health. This change is due to increased blood flow to the brain and hormone release. Getting physically fit and functioning on a stable and regular basis can have a positive effect on one's mental health and can offer many other advantages, such as the following. Physical activity has been linked with relieving symptoms of depression and anxiety.

Physical fitness improves their quality of life in patients with schizophrenia and to decrease the symptoms of schizophrenia. Being healthy will make one's self-esteem higher. Working out can improve mental alertness and reduce fatigue—increased opportunities for social interaction, allowing improved social competencies.

How to Stay Fit After 50

There are some effective ways to stay fit after age 50, however difficult it may seem. These five tips can help you get fit when you are 50 years old and above.

Lift Weights

For older women, weight lifting can be the best way to maintain overall fitness and stop the slow creeping gain in fat. It is possible to develop strength with weight training at any age, and some studies published in 2009 show women building substantial muscle in their 70s by lifting weights 2 to 3 days a week.

Walk Regularly

Walking has repeatedly been shown to enhance cardiovascular fitness, help keep weight under control, and improve mood in those who maintain a daily walking routine. 2 Any aerobic exercise (cycling, jogging, and swimming) is excellent to maintain lower levels of body fat and improve strength and overall body tone, but after age 50, walking has some benefits. Walking offers unique advantages for older exercisers. The risk of injury is small, needs little equipment, can be done alone or in a group, and is easy to do on the way. Walking also helps to improve the protection of the joints and bones. Walking may be the most significant benefit is that it's useful. Walking for errands, giving your pet exercise, socializing, or getting out in the fresh air are all additional benefits of using a walking routine to keep fit? Combining walking with weight training and getting in shape after age 50, you will have a simple and effective way to get and keep.

Incorporate High-Intensity Interval Training (HIIT)

Training at intervals is a great way to improve health overall. It's quick and efficient, but it can be challenging. Start slowly and stop when you're winded, to get the benefits of interval training and minimize risk. If you're out walking, for example, increase your speed for 30 seconds and then return to your regular pace. Repeat that burst of 30 seconds once every 5 minutes. Go on until five, 30-second bursts are done.

You can find that as the days and weeks go by, you want to jog in that 30-second interval. The benefit of interval training is that you're in charge of commitment and amount of reps. although you are not in outstanding condition, you can add some high-intensity interval training and turn it up a notch. When beginning intervals, always look out for any warning signs if you overdo it.

Perform Core Exercises

Core exercise is often one of the first things to decline as we age and become less healthy. Weak core strength due to poor body mechanics and poor alignment can lead to a domino effect of other physical aches and pains.3 Sore back, hips, knees and necks can often be traced back to poor core strength. The core muscles contain more than just the stomach, so a regular core strength routine is crucial to carry out regularly. Do a strong 20-minute core workout 3 to 4 times a week to maintain the core strength and stability. Some great ways to strengthen your core muscles are to do simple exercises on body weight that cause the core to contract while you stabilize your body.

Eat Enough Protein

Many older women don't get enough protein to maintain muscle mass.4 Protein is the body's major building block, and it needs to be replenished regularly because it isn't stored. Protein may either be complete (those that contain eight essential amino acids) or incomplete (those that lack essential amino acids). Full proteins are present in most animal sources such as meat, fish, and eggs, while incomplete proteins are usually found in plants, fruits, and nuts.

Vegan and strict vegetarian athletes often struggle to get adequate protein if they don't pay close attention to the way the food sources are mixed. 5 If you don't get enough protein, muscle building, or maintenance may be difficult.

If you're a vegan, learning how to get enough of the essential nutrient is even more important to you. You should get and keep in shape after 50, but to get the most out of your exercise requires regular movement and a bit of knowledge.

Five Simple Tips for Women to Stay Fit After 50

As the years go by, many women find that, in their 40s and 50s, the lifestyle that succeeded in their 20s and 30s struggles to achieve the same results. When women enter their 50s (the average age of menopause onset), they will have to make up for changes in hormonal, cardiovascular, and muscle rates. In aged women, weight gain is normal due to reductions in muscle mass, accumulation of excess fat, and a lower metabolic rate of rest. Hormonal changes can cause a range of symptoms and increase the overall risk of heart and stroke disorders. And certain nutrient absorption can decrease as a result of a loss of stomach acid. Clearly, at age 50, your diet will look a little different from your previous diet. The aim of the "50 and over" diet is to maintain weight, eat heart-healthy foods, and stay strong above all! To live your 50s in great shape, use the following five tips.

1. Add B12 to your daily supplements

B12 protects healthy blood cells and nerves and is needed to make DNA. B12 is found mainly in fish and meat. When we age, our stomach acid reduces, making nutrients such as B12 more difficult to consume. Older adults are at higher risk of B12 deficiency, but adding a vitamin to your diet in an additional form (either by pill or shot) may help avoid symptoms— which can take years to appear — before they begin.

2. Really cut back on salt

The older we get, the more likely we will experience hypertension (high blood pressure) because, as we age, our blood vessels will become less elastic.

Having high blood pressure puts us in danger of stroke, heart attack, heart failure, kidney disease, and early death. In the American diet, about 72 percent of salt comes from processed foods. You should reduce your consumption of processed foods (chips, frozen dinners, canned soup, etc.) considerably and ideally forget about 1500 mg or less of sodium per day, which is about 1/2 tsp. When you cook at home, you should start adding flavorful herbs instead of oil. Some herbs also provide anti-cancer benefits; oregano, thyme, and rosemary all have high antioxidant content. Ditching processed food also means eating more whole foods like whole grains, fruits, and vegetables. This will increase the consumption of your fiber. Fiber helps you stay fuller longer, ensuring you can eat less all day long and be more likely to keep your weight going. Salt in foods you wouldn't expect can be "hidden."

3. Check your multivitamin for Iron

The average woman experiences menopause and finishes her menstrual period around the age of 50 years. The need for iron after menopause decreases to about 8 mg of iron a day. Although the body can't live without iron, an overabundance can also be dangerous. Iron toxicity can occur because iron is not excreted naturally by the body; too much can cause damage to the liver or heart and even death. Postmenopausal women should only be taking iron supplements as prescribed by a doctor. If there is iron in your multivitamin, then replace it.

4. Pay more attention to vitamin D and calcium

Because of improvements in gastric and hormones, D levels and calcium absorption tanks around age 40. Furthermore, evidence shows that postmenopausal women are at an increased risk of osteoporosis due to their lack of estrogen. And make matters worse, the body breaks down more bone after 50 than it builds up.

This puts women over 50 at risk for bone fractures and osteoporosis. It's ideal for eating adequate calcium before age 30, but it's never too late to increase your diet's rich calcium sources. Sardines, spinach, broccoli, and low-fat or fat-free milk and yogurt are fabulously rich sources of calcium. Additionally, your doctor should test your vitamin D levels and provide additional supplementation as needed (the calcium absorption requires vitamin D).

5. Eat like a Greek!

Our blood vessels are becoming less elastic as we age, and the force of blood flowing through our veins is becoming more significant. It puts women in menopause at an elevated risk for heart disease. Our risk— and that's delicious! Having a Mediterranean cruise when you retire is a great release of the stress, but shifting to a Mediterranean diet might be a better idea.

The Benefits of Exercise over 50

Staying fit can be overwhelming-especially as there are so many kinds of workouts and activities to choose from. You should never have to worry about calling backup. "To find fitness professional, you trust. Trainers who are typically specialized in corrective exercise and functional movement will have a lot of experience with 50 or older clients.

It keeps your mind sharp. Regular exercise over 50 years of age enhances cognitive function, including memory.

It improves your mental health. Far from having only physical benefits, taking the time to exercise can also boost psychological well-being dramatically.

It can help maintain muscle and bones. Incorporating strength training into the fitness routine is important in slowing down the loss of aging muscle mass.

Maintaining active is also important for your bones, as maintaining bone density can reduce the risk of falling. It can lower the risk of certain diseases.

Regular physical activity can reduce the risk of heart disease, certain types of cancer, and developing diabetes. Regular exercise avoids many of the age-related medical problems, including developing type II diabetes and insulin resistance. It can help prevent and manage high blood pressure, type II diabetes, and high cholesterol. These all contribute to cardiovascular disease like heart attacks and strokes. Exercise must be part of your routine and must be performed 5-6 days a week. "When questioned about balancing exercise and diet to reduce the risk of developing medical problems," If you combine regular exercise with a careful diet, it's one of the easiest ways to minimize the number of drugs you need to take when you grow older.

1.3 Stay Active with Incidental Exercise

It can be daunting to try to stay fit after 50 when your definition of exercise is just those heart-pounding, high-energy workouts. There are many different things that count as an activity you have probably not even thought of. Things such as moderate housework (such as sweeping and vacuuming), gardening, ballroom dancing, and canoeing also help to raise your heart rate and benefit your health.

1. Go to Group Fitness Classes

One of the good ways to get motivated to work out is to sign up for a group fitness class. Many studios even offer free or discounted trial times, making it easy to find out where you feel most comfortable and what kinds of workouts you enjoy. You'll get into a routine after you start attending classes regularly— and perhaps even make some new friends along the way.

2. Eat more Plant-Based Meals

Staying fit means filling your body with healthy foods that improve your health and well-being— and evidence suggests the best possible plant-based sources. Having found that adhering to a plant-based diet will reduce your risk of heart failure by more than 40%. So avoid processed meat and sugar and instead fill your plate full of fruit, vegetables, whole grains, and protein-dependent on plants.

3. Chat with your Doctor about Your Fitness

Regular doctor appointments help your health during every stage of your life, but keeping up with them in your 50's is especially important. "Sure, you'll talk to your doctor about heart health and fitness," a trainer at Everybody Fights boxing gym. "We will let you know exactly what you can and can't do based on your current health and any medications that you may be on."

4. Track Your Steps

One of the best ways to stay fit after 50 is to make sure that during the day, you're getting around enough. Invest in a fitness tracker that will monitor your steps and make it your task to reach your target every day. Females in excess of 50 should take 10,000 steps a day, and men in excess of 50 should walk 11,000 to control their weight and be healthier overall.

5. Cut Back on Salt

It's hard to resist super-salty snacks, but it's time to start exercising a little more self-control, as you get older, because of the changing blood vessels you are more likely to develop high blood pressure. Which puts you at higher risk from a stroke and heart attack to kidney disease and death for everything? To reduce your risk of high blood pressure, cut salt— especially the high levels of sodium in processed foods— so that you can remain fit and healthy for years to come.

6. Don't Forget to Warm Up

It's just as necessary to warm up as your workout. Before each workout, it is essential to do one to get your blood flowing and to raise your heart rate. This can be as easy as walking on the treadmill, doing some jumping jacks, or going on a quick jog around the block— whatever helps relax the body and prepare for the workout.

7. Don't Limit Yourself to Cardio

This is not the only way to stay fit if you hate cardio — not by a long shot. It wasn't until we incorporated strength training that they began seeing and feeling the benefits of the time they spent in the gym. "James said that resistance training would help improve the balance, control blood sugar, develop bone density,

8. Drink Enough Water

Only think of water as the fuel for your body. If you don't get enough, how should this be working correctly? Water helps maintain the temperature in your body, preserving delicate tissues, lubricating and cushioning your joints, and helping with digestion— all items that you might need extra help as you age. For men, that means getting at least 3.7 liters of fluids a day, and for women, that means 2.7 liters of fluids a day — more so when you're exercising, since you need to replace lost fluids.

9. Always Focus on Form

You support your health as long as you have the exercise done, right? Ok, without proper form, you are not going to do any good. If you don't do the exercises correctly, you might put yourself at risk for injury that will only slow you down. If that means dabbing heavy dumbbells for lighter ones so you can better execute the motions, that are what needs to be done. You will develop the muscles and tone them, and be stronger in the process.

10. Start an Exercise Program

If you don't already have a solid exercise routine, it may be a good idea to kick things off with a structured workout program— something that will give you an action plan and detail what to do every day and for how long. That way, you're going to remain driven and have something to drive you. Exercising will become a routine by the time the program is over. There are plenty of different online choices to choose from depending on your favorite workout, whether it's a bodyweight exercise, dance, yoga, or a variety, so you're never going to get bored.

11. Keep a Food Journal

Your stomach, in your youth, cannot always do what it used to do. That's why keeping track of what you're eating — at least for a while, is essential. If you have a better understanding of what to put on your plate— and what to avoid!—It will boost your workouts, how you look, and your overall health throughout the day.

12. Have a "why" in Mind

It's hard to stick to anything unless the heart is in it. Once you start your journey of staying fit, make sure you know your "why." Maybe it's long enough around to see your grandchildren grow up, or maybe you want to be well enough to travel the world after retirement. Whatever the case may be, having a justification for what you are doing will help you stick to that dedication and sustain it as a top priority in your life.

13. Don't Push yourself too Hard

If you are still a fitness newbie, don't drive yourself too hard too quickly. Start gradually and ease your way into an exercise regimen that works for you, rather than rushing into the routine of intense full force, instead of jumping into an extreme full force routine.

By doing so, you're not only going to help prevent injuries and burnout, but you're also going to do some exercise you're looking forward to— not something you're dreading about.

14. Don't be Afraid to Make Changes

If something isn't working with your workout routine, don't be afraid to make any changes. But if it doesn't help you reach your goals or you don't like it, it might be the way to find out what's best for you and your body (yes, even if it means you cancel your gym membership by joining a yoga studio instead).

15. Utilize Online Workout Videos

Although many online fitness programs and subscription services cost money, going to YouTube alone will get you fit at no cost. There are countless quantities of fitness videos that inspire you to exercise right in the comfort of your home, including all-level yoga flows, high-intensity training sessions, low-impact mat-based exercises, mood-boosting Zumba classes, and more! Essentially, you're able to find something that concerns you.

16. Focus on Low-Impact Exercise

You don't want to do anything that is going to cause injury or pain when you're in your 50s. For this cause, James is a big fan of low-impact workouts. They're a great way to ease up your workout routine— especially if you haven't been up to one before. Activities such as walking, dancing, Pilates, and tai chi are all great possibilities.

17. Become a Yogi

Yoga is indeed the best way to stay active no matter what your age is. The yoga asanas are an amazing way to achieve the highest level of flexibility as well as relaxation in life.

There are many types of yoga that you can choose from to see which one fits you according to your current level of flexibility and agility.

18. Try Pilates

Pilates is one of the best moves with low impact to add to your workout routine. It is also gentle enough to help you heal from injuries and to prevent them, despite being a rigorous workout. It can help improve your posture, reduce pain, boost your flexibility and balance, and increase your endurance, as well as strengthening your muscles, taking classes, or doing online videos with the right form.

19. Make it Enjoyable

You won't stick to them if you dislike the workouts. For your best friends, you can love to run or lift weights, but if that isn't you, turn things up. You will stick with it for a long time to come when you find something that enhances your endorphins and makes you feel good.

20. Go for a Dip

Swimming is one of the most successful things you'll be doing in your fifties. It works all over your body, and because of its low impact, it protects your joints from stress and strain. The chance of early death for swimmers is 28 percent lower. What's more, being in and around the water can help you alleviate built-up stress and tension, which can affect your mental health.

21. Get a Workout Planner

It may feel stupid to have a separate calendar just for your workouts, but it may be the key to helping you stay in good shape all your life.

Identify exactly how you're going to stay healthy every day of the week every Sunday, whether you're doing it with an online video, heading to your favorite Pilates class, or walking on a nearby trail. This will help you keep track of what you're doing, and make sure you're not skipping your routine.

22. Walk as Much as You Can

It is easy to get lazier as you get older. Rather than walking the two blocks to the supermarket, you agree that just driving is a better idea. Okay, bring the car keys down. Consider it one of your top priorities every day to be more involved in every possible way. One of the most natural things to do is make sure you walk whenever possible

23. Connect with Nature

There's no fun being co-opted all day in a dreary gym. If it's nice out, take some time to exercise a few days a week in the great outdoors— whether you're walking around your neighborhood or hiking some trails in the woods. Outdoor exercise can provide a wide range of health benefits, including stress reduction, mood-boosting and self-esteem, and enhanced physical fitness. It is the all-around winner.

24. Use a Vibration Plate

If you haven't already used the vibration plate in your local gym, you'll want to start right now. This workout-enhancing system transmits energy as it vibrates to your body, which in turn causes your muscles to relax and contract several times per second. It can bring severe benefits for as little as 15 minutes of bodyweight exercises per day on the plate. "It has been shown to improve the growth of bone and muscle in older people. It could also help with weight loss and increasing strength.

25. Do Weight-Bearing Exercises

You don't have to go crazy about the weights to get your muscles working.

All you need is a pair of tiny dumbbells and some dedication. "Engage in weight-bearing exercise at least three days a week." We can just use a few light weights to help keep the muscle and bone.

26. Try Tai Chi

Tai chi is one of the good forms of exercise you can do, making it a top choice for all ages as well as fitness. Smooth, fluid movements not only help your body develop physically by improving your muscle strength and shape, flexibility, and balance. In essence, they also increase your energy levels and mood, as well as decrease tension, anxiety, and depression.

27. Improve your Gut Health

The nerves and muscles in your digestive tract may not function as well as they did in your fifties, resulting in issues such as constipation and diarrhea. Start offering your gut what it needs to thrive to keep feeling your best: probiotic supplements or fermented foods, choices such as sauerkraut and kombucha will increase the number of healthy bacteria in your gut, enhancing your overall micro biome. You'll have more time, feel happier, and like a champ, you can power through your workouts and the to-do list.

28. Stretch your Muscles Regularly

Stretching is never the top priority list of anyone, but it is just as important as working out. "As we age, our strength decreases and tight or weak muscles make you susceptible to injury and pain (especially with your knees and lower back), so take the time to stretch after any workout," James says. "Any simple static stretch— likes, for example, a hamstring stretch — should last about 30 seconds."

29. Work out with a Friend

Find a partner to make it more fun. Maybe it's someone you've met in one of your group fitness classes, a co-worker or family friend.

Whatever it may be, plan regular walks, yoga sessions, or whatever you both enjoy. It's the perfect double-whammy: time with someone you love to be around and get your sweat on.

30. Get your Protein Fix

Since you lose muscle naturally as you age, getting adequate protein through diet is crucial to your health and wellbeing. In addition to regular exercise, Nutrition has found that getting enough protein each day can help in reversing muscle loss. Select heart-sanitary choices such as lentils and legumes, almonds, quinoa, wild rice, tempeh, and tofu.

31. Do a Weight-Loss Challenge

If in your 50s, one of your primary reasons for getting fit is weight loss. There are even ways in which you can make things more fun, such as using Diet Bet, which helps you to win money as you shed pounds. You can put your target weight on a dry-erase board as well, and cross the pounds until you hit it.

32. Allow Time for Recovery

Exercise will take more of a toll on your body as you get older. Recovery time is very critical in taking full advantage of all the positive changes that occur in your body after a workout, to make sure you're ready for your workouts. That means staying hydrated, adding carbs and protein to your meals, and getting enough sleep to heal and feel the best you can.

33. Focus on your Rest

In recovery, sleep is not just important— it's essential in everything. When you age, you can experience more sleep problems— such as insomnia or snoring —but having enough rest is so important to your health and stay fit. Seek to get your immune system working correctly between seven and nine hours a night, help grow muscle and heal tissues, and synthesize hormones.

In the Sleep Department, if you cut yourself short, you'll feel it in more ways than one.

34. Balance Heavy Workouts with Light Ones

Another part of the process of healing is to make sure you match severe, sweat-dripping workouts with lighter ones. Instead of continually doing high-energy exercises that leave you tired and sore, it's best to add a few low-impact workouts— such as light yoga, jogging, or stretching-based sessions— to your routine too. Physically, you'll feel better, have better blood flow, and help relieve any muscle tightness you're feeling.

35. Find a Personal Trainer

If you believe an expert would better guide you through your workouts, try a personal trainer. It also ensures that you do every exercise correctly and that you develop a good form that can strengthen your body.

36. Work on Your Posture

If you have slacked on good posture over the years, now is the time to start paying more attention to your body alignment, standing up straight helps reduce discomfort by avoiding pressure on your joints, muscles, and spine. It can also boost your mood, lower your risk of injury, and help improve your workouts and strengthen your muscles.

37. Use Resistance Bands

Small dumbbells are a great way to keep fit; Paulvin also recommends band-based workouts for resistance. With any muscle group in your body, it is a gentle way to work — especially because the bands come in different strengths, depending on your current fitness level. And they're easy to pack up and take along on your trips while you're traveling.

38. Take in Some Vitamin-D

Vitamin D plays an important part in your health, particularly with your bones. You might need to increase the amount of osteoporosis, splits, and fractures that you get as you age. While supplements may help keep your levels healthy, doctors also advise you to stay active. Since the sun is a great source, ten to fifteen minutes of sunlight can also help keep you safe on your arms and legs a few days a week.

39. Start Resistance Training

If you have not applied to your routine resistance training — which involves working against your body weight or using dumbbells and exercise machines— start now? "It's going to help with your balance, muscle loss, and overall health. Even starting small with a few sessions a week will make you feels different.

40. Make Time for Meditation

When it comes to staying fit in your 50s, it is just as important to take care of your mind as taking care of your body. Regular meditation can help reduce anxiety, depression, and stress, as well as help, reduce pain, improve quality of life, reduce inflammation, and increase immune response. It's something that strengthens you from head to toe that you should do every day — even for just 10 minutes.

41. Don't do anything that Hurts

Though some exercises may feel great, others may not. "If what you're doing hurts, stop right away," — even if you're in a class surrounded by others. Always go with the workouts that make the body feel healthy instead of sticking with something uncomfortable just because you feel like you've gotta. Alternatively, this could result in an accident that will prevent you from achieving your goals.

42. Improve your Mobility

One way to talk about accidents is to work on improving your mobility — meaning your ability to move freely and easily. "This will help not only your endurance but also your cognitive ability to execute a movement that produces a strong body properly," she says. There are many different ways you can do this, such as through hip openers and half-circles in the back. It all depends on which areas you should be working on.

43. Limit your Alcohol Intake

Now and then, you might like to have a drink, but don't make it a regular occurrence. As you grow older, your body's alcohol tolerance lowers, which makes you feel its effects faster and puts you at a higher risk for accidents and injuries. Drinking can also lead to more health problems. Instead, stick to mostly water, tea, and other healthy fluids to ensure you feel your best throughout your 50s and beyond.

44. Zone in on your Back Muscles

It's essential to keep the back healthy as you age. Dedicate 15 minutes a day to a variety of exercises that can help prevent any complications happening in your back, including knee-to-chest stretches, bridges, and cat stretches.

45. Focus on the Small Things

Don't just focus on getting your fitness journey to those big goals. Focusing on the smaller milestones along the way is one way to enjoy the trip too. "It doesn't matter if you're doing a 5K or 10 push-ups with no rest, give yourself something to strive for, these achievements that feel small right now, but they're significantly improving your health.

46. Find a Good Playlist

It's not fun for anyone to work out in silence. If you want to make, your workout fly through — and enjoy every second that you sweat it out! — to concentrate on the song. "While you're working out, always listen to your favorite music. This makes a huge difference in your mood, and when you're feeling happy and positive, your workouts will also go well.

47. Try Cold Laser Therapy

When you think it takes you a long time to recover from exercise, one thing that could help is to use cold laser therapy to help with aches and pains. "People who practice or continue to play sports in their 50s can retain strength and endurance. The downside is that it takes their bodies far longer to recover," "Whole-body cold laser therapy, like Prism Light Pod, will help speed up recovery four to ten times faster."

48. Try Red Light Therapy

Red light therapy is known to help with everything from clearer skin and fewer wrinkles to increase hair growth. One thing people don't realize is it's nice to stay fit in your older years too. "Red light therapy has been demonstrated to encourage bone growth, improve testosterone in men, and help maintain thyroid." This should be performed three to five days a week.

Chapter 2: Best ways to weight loss for women after 50

2.1 20 Tips for Weight Loss

To many women, it can become harder to maintain a healthy weight or lose excess body fat as the years go by. Unhealthy habits, a lifestyle that is mostly sedentary, poor food choices, and metabolic improvements, can all contribute to weight gain after age 50. Nevertheless, you can lose weight at any age with a few quick changes-regardless of your physical abilities or medical diagnoses.

There are 20 best ways to lose weight after 50.

1. Learn to Enjoy Strength Training

While cardio gets a lot of attention when it comes to weight loss, strength training is also important for older adults in particular. Your muscle mass decreases as you age, in a process called sarcopenia. This muscle mass loss begins around the age of 50 and can slow down metabolism, which can lead to weight gain. Your muscle mass decreases by around 1–2 percent per year after age 50. When the muscle strength decreases at a rate of 1.5–5percent per annum. To that age-related muscle loss and promote a healthy body weight, adding muscle-building exercises to your routine is therefore necessary. Strength training, such as exercises on body weight and weightlifting, will significantly improve muscle strength and increase muscle size and function. However, strength training will help you lose weight by reducing body fat and increasing your metabolism, which will improve the number of calories you consume during the day.

2. Team up

It can be challenging to put in a healthy eating pattern or workout routine on your own. Pairing with a friend, coworker, or family member may give you a better chance to stick to your plan and achieve your goals for wellness. Evidence, for example, indicates that those completing weight loss programs with friends are considerably more likely to sustain their weight loss over time. Living with friends can also affirm your dedication to a fitness program and make the workout more enjoyable.

3. Sit Less and Move More

Burning more calories is key to removing excess body fat than you take in. That's why it is essential to be more active all day while trying to lose weight.

Sitting at your job for long periods, for example, could hinder your attempts to lose weight. To combat this, simply by getting up from your office and taking a five-minute walk every hour, you can become more involved in the job. Using a pedometer or fit bit to monitor your steps will improve weight loss by increasing your activity levels and calorie consumption. Start with a practical step goal based on your current level of activity when using a pedometer or Fit bit. Then work your way steadily up to 7,000–10,000 steps per day or more depending on your overall health.

4. Bump up your Protein Intake

It is not only necessary for weight loss to get enough high-quality protein in your diet but also essential to avoid or reverse age-related muscle loss. Eating a diet high in proteins, however, will help prevent or even reverse muscle loss. Increasing protein in the diet can help you lose weight and keep it off in the long run. Older adults have greater protein needs than younger adults, so adding protein-rich foods to your meals and snacks is even more important

5. Talk to a Dietitian

Finding an eating pattern that both encourages weight loss and feeds on the body can be challenging. Consulting a licensed dietitian will help you find out how best to lose excess body fat without taking an overly restrictive diet. Furthermore, a dietitian will help and direct you on your path to weight loss. Meeting with a dietitian to lose weight will lead to significantly better results than going to it yourself, and over time it can help you keep the weight loss down.

6. Cook more at Home

Those who cook and consume more home-made meals tend to have a healthier diet and weigh less than those who do not. Cooking meals at home allows you to monitor what's going into your recipes— and what's left out. It also helps you to play with good, special. This also lets you play with fine, unique ingredients that interest you. When you take the bulk of meals outside the building, start cooking at home for one or two meals a week, then slowly increase the number until you cook more than you eat out at home.

7. Eat more Produce

Vegetables and fruits are filled with vital nutrients for your wellbeing, and adding them to your diet is an easy, evidence-based way to minimize excess weight. For example, a study of 10 studies found that each daily rise in vegetable serving was correlated with a 0.14-inch (0.36-cm) reduction in female waist circumference. Another research in 26,340 men and women aged 35–65 led to eating fruits and vegetables lower in body weight, decreased waist circumference, and less body fat.

8. Hire a Personal Trainer

In particular, training with a personal trainer will help someone new to working out by showing you the best way to exercise to encourage weight loss and avoid injury.

Plus, you may be motivated by personal trainers to work out more by keeping you accountable. They can even improve your workout behavior. A 10-week study in 129 adults revealed that one-on-one personal training for 1 hour per week increased exercise motivation and increased levels of physical activity.

9. Rely Less on Convenience Foods

Eating convenience foods daily, such as fast food, candy, and fried snacks, is associated with weight gain and may impede your efforts to lose weight. Convenience foods tend to be high in calories and low in important nutrients such as fat, sugar, vitamins, and minerals. This is why fast foods and other processed foods are widely referred to as "empty calories." A good way to lose weight is to cut back on fried foods and substitute them with balanced meals and snacks revolving around nutrient-dense whole foods.

10. Finding an Activity, You Enjoy

It can be difficult to find an exercise routine that you can sustain over the long term. That is why participating in the activities this you enjoy is significant. If solo activities are more of your style, try your bike, cycle, hike, or swim.

11. Get Checked by a Healthcare Provider

If you are struggling to lose weight while being active and keeping a balanced diet, disorders that can make it difficult to lose weight, such as hypothyroidism and polycystic ovarian syndrome (PCOS), maybe justifiable to rule out. It can be particularly valid if you have members of your family with those conditions. Tell your healthcare professional about your symptoms so that they can agree on the best testing procedure to rule out medical problems that might be behind your weight loss struggles.

12. Eat a Whole-Foods-Based Diet

One of the good ways to ensure the body gets the nutrients it needs to survive is by having an adequate diet in whole food. Whole foods, including vegetables, fruits, seeds, nuts poultry, fish, legumes, and grains, are filled with nutrients that are important to maintaining healthy body weight, such as fiber, calcium, and healthy fats, whole-food diets, both plant-based and animal-based diets, have been associated with weight loss.

13. Eat Less at Night

Eating fewer calories at night will help keep your bodyweight safely and lose excess body fat. A survey of 1,245 people found that those who consumed more calories at dinner over six years were more than two times more likely to become obese than those who eat more calories earlier in the day. Additionally, those who ate more calories at dinner were considerably more likely to develop metabolic syndrome, a category of disorders involving high blood sugar and excess belly fat. Metabolic syndrome increases your risk of developing heart disease, diabetes, and stroke. Eating most of your calories during breakfast and lunch, while having a lighter dinner, maybe a good weight loss process.

14. Focus on Body Composition

Though bodyweight is a good health measure, your body composition-meaning the percentages of fat and fat-free mass in your body is also significant. Muscle mass, especially in older adults, is an important measure of overall health. The target should be to pack on more muscle and shed excess fat. There are many ways to measure the proportion of your body fat. Measuring your hips, biceps, calves, chest, and thighs will help you determine if you lose fat and gain muscle.

15. Hydrate the Healthy Way

Beverages such as sweetened coffee beverages, soda, juices, sports drinks, and premade smoothies are often filled with calories and added sugars. Drinking sugar-sweetened beverages are strongly linked to weight gain and conditions such as obesity, heart disease, diabetes, and fatty liver disease, particularly those sweetened with high-fructose corn syrup. Swapping sugar beverages with nutritious drinks such as water and herbal tea can help you lose weight, and can substantially reduce your risk of developing the above described chronic conditions.

16. Choose the Right Supplements

If you feel tired and unmotivated, taking the right supplements may help you get the energy you need to achieve your goals. Your ability to absorb those nutrients decreases and the risk of deficiencies are increasing. For example, adults over 50 are typically deficient in folate and vitamin B12, two nutrients needed to produce energy. Deficiencies in B vitamins such as B12 can adversely affect your mood, cause fatigue, and inhibit weight loss. For that reason, taking a high-quality B-complex vitamin to help lower the risk of deficiency is a good idea for those over the 50s.

17. Limit Added Sugars

Limiting high-added sugar foods, including sweetened beverages, sweets, cakes, cookies, ice cream, sweetened yogurts, and cereals, is key to weight loss at any age. Since sugar is added to so many foods, including things that you wouldn't expect like tomato sauce, salad dressing, and bread, the easiest way to determine if an item contains added sugar is to read ingredient labels. Look for "added sugars" on the label of nutrition facts, or check for popular sweeteners like cane sugar, high-fructose corn syrup, and agave ingredients list.

18. Improve your Sleep Quality

Does not get enough quality sleep will harm your efforts to lose weight. Failure to get enough sleep increases the likelihood of obesity and may impede attempts to lose weight. For example, a two-year study of 245 women showed that those who slept 7 hours a night or more were 33 percent more likely to lose weight compared to those who slept less than 7 hours per night, the better quality of sleep was also associated with success on weight loss.

19. Try out Intermittent Fasting

Intermittent fasting is a form of eating pattern in which you eat only for a given period of time. The most common form of intermittent fasting, followed by a 16-hour fast, is the 16/8 eating method within an 8-hour period. Intermittent fasts foster weight loss. However, some test-tube and animal studies indicate that intermittent fasting can benefit older adults by improving longevity, slowing down the decline of cells, and preventing age-related changes in your cells ' energy-producing sections of mitochondria.

20. Be more Mindful

Eating carefully can be an easy way to improve your food relationship, while at the same time promoting weight loss. Beware eating means paying more attention to your eating habits and food. It gives you a better understanding of your signs of hunger and fullness and how food affects your mood and wellbeing. Use conscientious eating strategies encourage weight loss, and eating habits improve. There are no specific rules for eating conscientiously, but eating slowly, paying attention to the scent and taste of each bite of food, and keeping track of how you feel during your meals are simple ways of adding careful eating to your life.

Another 14 Most Effective Ways to Lose Weight After 50

There's no excuse that at 50, you can't look as fit and glamorous as at 40, but there's one hitch: once they reach this landmark era, even stars with personal trainers and fitness coaches have to work a bit harder to lose the pounds. You'll have to put extra effort into one of the main reasons: your body composition changes as you age. For every ten years after age 35, you lose muscle mass at an average rate of 3-5 percent, and this can affect the way you burn fat. "The body is going through aging as it leaves the growing one.

Why it's harder to lose weight after 50

They take their toll all those years of playing sports, chasing after your family, and walking up and down stairways. You may note that your joints are a little stiffer than they were a few decades ago, and your muscles are a bit more sorry. Then, there's your ever-evolving metabolism problem. You are resting on the metabolic rate, the capacity of your body to burn fat while sitting on the sofa doing nothing decreases by around 1-2 percent per decade due to loss of muscle mass and increased fat mass. Generally, our diets don't change enough to compensate for this metabolic transition, ensuring that with every birthday weight will slowly but surely creep up. "There are a variety of roadblocks that people will face while trying to lose weight in their 50s," "But once you know what they are— and how to get around them— it's easy to succeed in falling pounds." One of the best things you can do at any age is to change your routine and try something new. Follow these tips to help you drop the pounds, and hold them off for good, courtesy of some of the best weight-loss experts, dietitians, and personal trainers in the country.

1. Talk to Your Doctor about a Weight-Loss Plan

First, stop after the big 5-0—your doctor's office celebrates. She can assess your current health status, address any health issues that might affect your weight (such as pre-diabetes or sleep apnea), and help you come up with a diet and exercise plan. She might even recommend you to a physiotherapist or personal trainer.

2. Get your Hormones Checked

Let her test your hormone levels while you are at the doctor's office. When we age, progesterone, testosterone, and other hormones are decreasing, which is setting the body up to store fat instead of weight loss. "Just monitoring the thyroid, adrenal glands, and other levels of hormones— and then taking the appropriate measures to get them back into balance — can go a long way towards helping people lose weight in their 50s," he said.

3. Set Realistic Goals

To announce that you will lose 20 pounds before next month's beach holidays is impractical, not to mention unhealthy. "Be honest with yourself. How are you feeling? How strong are you? Changing life requires bravery and mental strength. Divide big targets into smaller, more realistic ones. Instead of the number on the scale, focusing on how you feel and the positive changes you're making to your lifestyle will help you stay motivated to reach your goals. "Triumphs create your confidence. "Small successes lead to big goals accomplished." Middle Eastern meze platter of green falafel, pita, and sun-dried tomatoes, pumpkin and beet hummus, olives, stuffed peppers, tabouleh, figs. The idea for the Mediterranean appetizer group.

4. Consult a Dietitian

There are dozens of different food plans floating around the internet, each claiming to help you shed the pounds without feeling deprived (the Mediterranean Diet, the DASH Diet, and the WW Freestyle are some of the best diets for weight loss by 2020). An RD will also provide your suggestions on how to fix roadblocks that might interfere with your goals, such as emotional stress feeding, insulin intolerance, nutritional deficiencies, and meal-prep fatigue.

5. Follow a Structured Plan

By 50, you've had enough runs around the block to realize that the fad diets don't work. "No crazy fasts, no shaving, heavy cutting or complex carbohydrates or proteins. Unlock your genetic potential for the power, health, and beauty of the Ageless. Consider then adopting a clinically proven program that is controlled by medication. These types of applications, mainly if they include personal support and weekly check-ins, have a weight-loss success rate of more than 75%.

6. Embrace Strength Training

Even if in your life you've never picked up a dumbbell, now's the best time to learn how to use the weight room (but please, if you're a newbie, first work with a trainer, so you don't injure yourself!). Because the trick to losing weight over 50 is this: Create more muscle mass to boost your metabolism (you now have about 20 percent less than when you were 20). "The good news is that with a well-structured weight-training routine, you can turn all of this around." That can help you regain the ability to lose weight just as you were able to do 20 years ago. Get weights lifted at least twice a week, whether you are using free weights or equipment or doing bodyweight exercises. Rising every day doesn't hurt — just make sure you work for different muscle groups or exercise each day differently.

7. Choose Activities that are Easy on the Joints

Among her 50-somethings, she gets the best performance when she has them doing some cross-training in the pool. Weak knees can help prevent you from getting a great workout, and aches and pains can completely turn some people off exercise. "Water movement on the joints is simple and can also improve the range of motion." Much better, caloric expenditure is about 30 percent higher in water than on land because of the resistance that water produces. "No pool? No trouble. Walking is another popular aerobic activity with small impacts, such as running, kayaking, yoga, and dancing.

8. Make the Most out of Every Workout

When you try to block the moment, cram into your sports bra and get to the gym, don't let yourself. Exhaustion or sore joints prevent you from going all out. This is one of the 50-year-olds ' biggest pet peeves. "Far too many people think they're working out just because they showed up."

9. See a Physical Therapist

If a sore back, wonky knee or creaky hip has stopped you from regularly working out, make an appointment with a physical therapist. "For 50 years, many people have sustained injuries and don't know what their habits are. Getting advice from a doctor can help."

10. Overhaul your Diet

Just as pop music isn't the same as when you were in your 30s, so your metabolism has shifted too, meaning you eat about 250 fewer calories every day. So if you keep tasting as you did in the early 2000s — and don't raise your exercise — you will eventually rise in weight. Removing the junk food in your diet and replacing it with tons of fruits, vegetables, whole grains, and lean proteins will make it painless to cut calories.

11. Change How and when you eat

When planning your meals, the focus is on completeness and no portion control. "When it comes to a safe weight loss, then we want to strike the delicate balance between eating until we feel complete then fulfilled because our total calorie intake is always dropping."

12. Get your Stress in Check

Your 50s can be a prime time for tension between paying college tuition for your children, managing more and more obligations at work, and coping with the aging parents. The solution: plan your workouts as the appointments of a doctor. Not only can adhering to a daily schedule help relieve tension, but it can also help you stay on board with the diet. After all, who wants to eat a donut to spoil the benefits of a tough sweat session?

13. Get your Sleep

One great thing about being 50—you're entirely over the social pressure of staying out late. Doing everything you can to get 7-8 hours of snooze every night is key to helping you lose weight. During daily shut-eyes, the two hormones that control appetite— leptin, and ghrelin— go into overdrive. "This can cause excessive hunger at any age and lead to poor food choices and weight gain. Right here is a list of tested sleep strategies.

14. Practice Self-Care

Whether it's treating you to a manicure or taking a day off from work for mental health, taking care of yourself shouldn't be seen as a luxury. Smallest movements can make a big difference in stress reduction, which can significantly impact your weight loss. Furthermore, you can use that motivation to do things that support your goals, such as eating healthy, exercising, and meditating, if you give yourself a little more affection.

Not sure how to continue daily self-care? Then ask yourself why you need more time to get yourself cared for. Would you work too many hours late at the office? Did you feel stressed out, and want to be calmer? When you find out why you need to spend some more time on your own, it can help you decide what's going to be a good habit or routine.

2.2 The 5 Crucial Diet Changes Women Over 50 Must Make

The diet of a person after 50 is crucial. It is the most important factor, arguably, in maintaining a healthy body at this age. The side effects are imminent. Proper nutrition is essential throughout the entire lifespan, of course. Still, around and after age 50, changes take place inside the body that makes the food you eat of particular significance, "As you age, you lose muscle mass, around 10 percent every decade after age 50." "When you lose your muscle, you are more likely to gain body fat and need fewer calories "because the muscle consumes more calories than body fat. Prioritizing exercise is also essential — especially resistance training to help counteract the decline in metabolism that happens with aging. Nutrition must be given priority to avoid heart disease, diabetes, and other diseases that are of more significant concern as people grow older.

Eat: Fatty Fish

"Every week, having at least two 3.5-ounce servings of cooked fatty fish such as salmon, tuna, or herring will help keep your heart safe. These fish provide omega-3 fatty acids that support the heart. They are essential to the overall health of an individual and are promoted for their protective effects, especially on the brain, eyes, and heart.

Eat: Prunes

Bone health matters as you age. About one-third of women and 20 percent of men over the age of 50, due to osteoporosis, break a bone. "Eating prunes helps to reinforce bone health and keep the bones healthy." Also, she says, eating five to six prunes a day has been shown to help prevent bone loss, per Osteoporosis International research. "You can snack prunes, add them to a salad, or make preserves or even brownies with them."

Eat: Tomato Sauce

Surprisingly this diet is helping to reduce wrinkles. "Tomatoes are red gems which supply the antioxidant lycopene." She adds that this antioxidant can help protect the skin from wrinkles and other damage caused by UV light. Cooked tomatoes are preferred because your body better absorbs the lycopene. You may apply tomato sauce to the pasta, or use it in a recipe for spaghetti squash.

Limit: Added Sugars

All people will restrict the consumption of added sugar, and as you get older, this is even more important. "Added sugar like table sugar and brown sugar should constitute no more than 10% of your total calories. "That's about 12 teaspoons of added sugar for a 2,000-calorie daily diet. "I suggest using one which offers some nutrition for the added sugar that you add to your day. My favorite is pure maple syrup. "It's a rare sweetener because it contains 60-plus health-helping polyphenols, as well as mineral manganese and B vitamin riboflavin that aids in the blood. I like using it to sweeten grains overnight, a muffin recipe, or a maple-Dijon salad dressing."

Don't Eat: Trans Fats

While you always want to stop these, it's even more important to do so as you get older.

Estrogen provides an absolute defense against heart disease before menopause. "But women are at an increased risk of heart disease after menopause— and Trans fats don't support the situation. "You will boost your' weak' LDL cholesterol, lower your' healthy' HDL cholesterol, and increase the risk of heart disease." Prevent it by reading labels of ingredients to make sure the partially hydrogenated oil is not an ingredient.

Best Diets for Women Over 50

When women approach 50, their bodies plan for menopause and go through other side effects of aging. To order to maintain their health, many people need to follow new and different strategies, including changing their diets, to receive the required nutrients. We may want to look at the best foods for women over 50, in that case. "Thanks to perimenopause and menopause, the 50s are a time for significant changes. This is a time in the woman's life in which she has hormone variations, which can cause metabolism and body weight changes. Kay also mentions osteoporosis, osteoarthritis, and changes in the regulation of blood sugar (insulin resistance may occur as a result of changes in hormones) as other disorders women may encounter in this age group.

Mediterranean

The Mediterranean diet is healthy for heart health and can prevent diabetes and cancer. It does not limit or exclude certain food groups but instead promotes all in moderation. In addition to whole grains, it emphasizes fruit and vegetable carbohydrates, which have plenty of fiber and will leave you feeling full for longer. The Mediterranean diet stresses omega-3 fats found in olive oil and fish. This has plenty of omega-3 fats found in foods such as fish and olive oil, which also improve satiety in addition to aiding in hormone production. It is also rich in protein, in plant-and animal products. This protein is essential for women over 50 who need it to fight against muscle loss that happens with age.

Paleo

The Paleo diet is a low-carbohydrate, high-protein meal plan rich in vegetables, plants, fruits, nuts, and unprocessed meat. The lower level of carbohydrates is helpful for women in their 50s and older age that may have insulin resistance and are unable to absorb carbs like they were before. The Pale diet incorporates protein and reduces soy and dairy products. "Paleo does not have soy or milk that can help women with hormone changes because excess soy and hormones found in traditional dairy products can contribute to high levels of estrogen, The women store weight in their hips and thighs. "This also contains good fats to encourage the safe development of hormones.

Whole Foods

The whole real food diet, or "clean eating," excludes all processed foods that can reduce inflammation. This food can also help manage hormones due to the lack of antibiotics or preservatives in whole grains, which can be significant disruptors to the hormones. Packaged foods on a Whole Foods diet are not permitted. It focuses on all real food products, such as fruits, vegetables, legumes, whole grains, fish, meats, and healthy fats. The absence of processed food is equivalent to less refined sugars, resulting in better control of blood sugar and less accumulated abdominal fat. The high number of nutrients and fiber present in these foods often contributes to feeling full, avoiding overeating.

Autoimmune Protocol (AIP)

The autoimmune protocol (AIP) focuses on restoring the gut and reducing inflammation, which can be of great help to women in their 50s familiarity with the hormonal changes. It can also eliminate harmful foods and activate, such as refined sugars and processed foods, which can cause malabsorption and inflammation in the intestine.

Sugar fiends can benefit from the AIP diet, removing the sweet things. "If the gut is unsanitary, it will hinder the ability of the body to absorb nutrients. It creates hormonal imbalances that worsen the changes already occurring in the hormone." AIP also strengthens the immune system, which can reduce the risk of illness as we age.

Higher Protein/Moderate Carbohydrate

Eating food that is high in protein / moderate in carbohydrates will help the body during its natural aging cycle. Studies have found that higher levels of protein sustain the muscle mass of your body as it declines as you age and keep you full, reducing the amount of food that is eaten. It can help stabilize your blood sugar levels by raising your protein and lowering your carbohydrates.

Performing' fasted cardio' is one of the most effective ways to burn fat or keeps weight off. This practice includes cardio of any sort, whatever your level at any speed; first thing you've eaten in the morning before. It requires the body to supply all the energy since there is no food at all! Don't worry about hitting those weights also if you're starting slow and lighting its progress! Ladies tend to worry about getting nearer to weight training. They imagine rooms of pumped-up sweaty men grunting, and sadly sometimes this is true! (Or not unfortunately based on preference)

However the old rhetoric we'd drummed into us that weights make you bulky is a pure myth, women don't have the testosterone in their system to create large muscles, even if it would need very strong repeated poundage's, and vast amounts of bodybuilding dose protein intake too! Think that if a vehicle has four people inside, it uses more fuel than if it has one.

Heavier weight lifting burns up more calories than lightweight. And it usually does make you smaller.

In recent times, the old way of thinking that we can't eat after 8 pm or that we don't have carbs after 4 pm has proved wrong. Dinner carbohydrates also encourage the production of serotonin in the brain and help the sleep of a better night. We even keep us happier throughout the evening time when many of us start searching in cupboards dangerously! Fat doesn't make you greasy! We need to be much more preoccupied with sugar instead. Sugar causes an insulin spike, which prompts fat storage immediately. Check the back of what you're consuming and know a teaspoon is 5 g of sugar. When you eat a salad with 15 g of sugar in it, something is wrong! Make ALL protein-meals. Putting on weight is extremely difficult if that is the crux of your plan. Don't think about the source you're using too much; if you love lamb; don't think about chicken, its perfect scrambled eggs.

Overall weight the main arbiter will not be the scales. Sure, you can keep an eye on things, but what if you put your muscle on 2 kg and you lose 2 kg of fat? Scales show little difference, but there were beautiful improvements to yours. Note 2 kilograms of muscle over the entire body is not anything; but, even though you're doing nothing, the muscle needs calories to survive.

You are about to change your metabolism to become a fat consuming furnace! Only a few tweaks will make all the difference to your workout choices. Exercises that use more muscles consume more calories and, including legs and back, appear to reach the larger muscles.

Hiring a trainer to take you through these more complicated choices for only a few sessions can put you on a path to even greater success and be worth the money in the long run.(maybe you have one fewer bottle of wine a week to make up for it!!) Try to rope a friend into going with you, sometimes you can both get bitten by the bug and inspire each other when you see results.

You're both going to have good days and bad days, but you're more likely to be consistent and having fun with a friend there. Look at the fitness timetables and mix with your weights for variety in some free classes like spinning, boxing, Zumba whatever you want; do it! My last suggestion is to try to have fun! If you don't feel like going one night, then don't! If you don't go, unwell! Don't listen if people say it's best to go in the morning or evening. Go whenever it suits you, and the gym shouldn't fit the other way around in your life. Anything worth doing is simple, but persistence produces results, and you'll be amazed at how fantastic you feel after a month, and your figure's compliments never hurt!

2.3 Metabolism-Boosting Tips for Women

Losing weight after being 50 years old is no easy feat. At the end of a hard day, not only are sugar treats enticing, but your metabolism has probably taken a nose-dive too. From the age of 20, the metabolism is slowing by about 2 percent every decade. You can understand why by the time you reach middle age, the scale is creeping up more quickly. Yet all hope is not lost. There are several ways to improve your metabolism fast; including the easiest approach you can start today.

1. Drink your Morning Coffee

A big one is that morning habit. Coffee is a popular choice drink for those over 50 years of age. And there is good news for your metabolism if you enjoy each morning reaching for a cup. Coffee may be able to elevate the metabolic rate in the short term. Nonetheless, make sure you do not add cream or sugar to your coffee, as all those extra calories quickly add up.

2. Get Adequate Rest

Sleep is vitally important to your health. It seems pretty straightforward, but most of us don't get as much sleep as we need. Everyday Health estimates that those around the age of 50 need to sleep between seven and nine hours per night. And if you're over 65, between seven and eight people need you. Having insufficient sleep can lead to several metabolic problems. "It can cause you to consume fewer calories, lack control of appetite, and experience a rise in levels of cortisol, which stores fat.

3. Chew Gum

Placing pink chewing gum in her mouth. This little trick is revitalizing your metabolism. Feeling that in your day, you don't get enough movement? The simple act of gum chewing is a convenient way to revive your metabolism without even noticing it. Researchers found those who chewed sugar-free gum three 20-minute intervals a day saw a 5 percent increase in their metabolism. This was a small study, and without proper diet and exercise, probably won't make a huge difference, but still — it seems like something so simple can make a difference over the long run.

4. Don't Skimp on your Daily Protein Intake

Proper nutrition is one of the most successful ways to ensure that the metabolism moans rapidly "there's some evidence that older adults need more protein." This nutrient can help to minimize age-related muscle degeneration. So muscle helps maintain a good metabolic rate, and you want to make sure that when you get older, you get enough. If you enjoy carb-heavy cooking, try 30 grams per meal and more.

5. Try 15 Minutes of Yoga

Even a brief yoga session can help. Getting up every day and doing a few minutes of yoga is the perfect way to get your metabolism going at a fast pace. "First thing in the morning, it can increase the metabolic rate. And he especially recommends sun salutations, as they are great for improving strength and flexibility through a sequence of movements that flow together. You are going to exercise without even knowing it.

6. Try Moderate-Intensity Cardio instead of High-Intensity

Now, jumping squats and burpees may be all the rage — and they're sure to beat your heart to its full. But for those over 50, such movements on your joints can be incredibly difficult. The good news is that exercising at high-intensity intervals is not the only way to revive your metabolism. Exercises with a lower impact are just as good for you, and more affordable for more people. A brisk daytime stroll or a peaceful evening bike ride is perfect for the mind and body — and they do much more for you than you think.

7. Move your Body more Throughout the Day

A fit bit will help to keep you on track.

We know you're busy — but don't forget to shift if you're sitting at a desk for most of your day. A little more than usual, jumping around will improve your metabolism long after you're back to sitting down again. And since a simple "walk around the block will triple your metabolic rate," it will also do your body right to shake your legs out and do some arm circles every hour or so.

8. Stand Instead of Sitting Whenever Possible

Make a point to stand instead of sitting. To get your metabolism going, you don't need to do strenuous exercise — or any activity at all.

Only standing for a few hours a day instead of sitting can provide you with multiple health benefits, "we don't have to use any muscles while we're sitting." So even standing more can improve your metabolism.

9. Drink Cold Water

Coldwater will increase metabolism. Used to drink your room temperature water? It may be in your interest to add a few ice cubes to your drink. Drinking 48 ounces of cold water a day can boost your metabolism enough to burn an additional 50 calories. That doesn't seem like much-but with minimal effort on your part; it can make a difference over time.

10. Avoid Diet Drinks

If you are going to be drinking soda, miss the diet variety, at least. It's getting harder to prevent the scale from creeping as you age — so you can settle for a soda diet or two during the day. But this is discouraged for the sake of your metabolic health. It is inconclusive; however, whether it is the diet soda or other elements of your diet that may be the more significant issue.

11. Eat More Eggs

Eggs represent a great source of protein. If eggs are your favorite protein, you are in luck. Not only do eggs fill, but they also contain all the essential amino acids that can then be used by your body to keep your metabolism going. The publication states that a protein-filled diet will improve your metabolism by up to 100 calories a day, as proteins require more energy to break down in the body. And when you're over 50, you can make a giant difference by adding 100 calories a burned day.

12. Sip on Green Tea

Green tea has many benefits. In addition to the cold water, you should also make a few more cups of tea than usual. Studies self-explain show that green tea drinkers can burn up to an extra 100 calories per day. That's because of Catechins, an antioxidant that helps the metabolism. Not all green tea can give the crowd of over 50 either. Green tea drinkers may have a higher chance of being healthy, versatile, and self-sufficient in their lives.

13. Get enough Zinc in your Diet

All of those foods contain zinc. A multivitamin that captures anything may not do enough for your body. Prevention explains that zinc is essential to your thyroid since it helps to generate hormones that control your metabolism and keep your energy levels up. Not only that, but it can help keep rates of hunger in the bay too. Most post-menopausal women have a zinc deficiency, so eat a serving of shellfish, dark poultry meat, or beef every once in a while to get your fill.

14. Imagine Working out without ever entering the Gym

If you can't make that happen, imagine the workout. Can't come for a stroll outside? No trouble. There are more benefits of visualizing a sweat session than you thought. In reality, it can trick your body into believing that physical exercise strengthens it, thus burning more calories and boosting your metabolism

15. Lift more Weights

Lifting weights prevents muscle loss and helps with calories burning. You needn't be a bodybuilder to see the advantages of lifting weights.

This will not only combat age-related muscle loss, but it can also help you eat more calories during the day.

Self says that when you're at rest, muscle consumes three times as many calories as fat. And if you're not a massive exercise fan, you can change your workout by picking a pair of dumbbells and making it more fun.

If you like what you are reading, I invite you to see my books with similar topics. Thanks for your attention and happy reading!

https://www.amazon.com/Dylan-Bold/e/B086N2WJYV

Chapter 3: Fitness and Exercise for Women

3.1 Get-Fit Advice for Women Over 50

Before 50, if you were physically active, this is perfect. But if you haven't been exercising regularly, starting is not too late. Physical activity can help to relieve some of the menopause symptoms— hot flashes, joint pain, and sleep problems. Additionally, it helps to control weight and absorbs fat in the belly. The effects of exercise are so strong that each physiological system in the body is affected for the better.

For those of you who have purchased the book or the audiobook, the exercises mentioned here and their references are attached in a PDF file that'll help you in carrying out the exercises.
You may ask for this pdf, by sending an email to "dylan.bold.author@gmail.com".
Staying Fit as You Age

There are many aging problems related to an inactive lifestyle. And while your chronological age maybe 55, if you adopt a regular exercise program, your biological age maybe 35-- Check with your doctor before you start, particularly if you have any of the heart disease risk factors (smoking, high blood pressure, high cholesterol, diabetes or family history). Then, move on.

Aerobic Exercise

Any type of cardiovascular conditioning is aerobic exercise. It may include such things as brisk walking, swimming, biking, or cycling. You probably know it as "cardio." By definition, aerobic exercise means "with oxygen." During aerobic exercises, breathing and heart rate will increase. Aerobic exercise helps maintain a healthy heart, lungs, and circulatory system. Aerobic exercise is distinct from that of anaerobic exercise. Anaerobic activities such as weight-lifting or sprinting involve rapid energy bursts. They're performed for a short time with maximum effort.

In contrast to aerobic exercises, this is. Aerobic exercises are performed for a sustained period. They can do cardiovascular exercises at home. With little to no equipment, there are many that you can do too. Warm-up always 5 to 10 minutes before any activity starts.

Jump Rope

Jumping rope helps build better body awareness, coordination with the hand-foot, and agility. Your jumping rope should be height adjustable. Stand with both feet on the center of the rope, and add the handles to your axes. That is the height that you're going for. If it is too long, cut or tie it so as not to get stuck onto the rope. Walking a jump rope circuit is a high indoor or outdoor sport, though you'll want to make sure you've got plenty of space. To complete your circuit routine, this should take 15 to 25 minutes.

Start by jogging forward by throwing the jumping rope over your head and under your feet. Make a move within 15 seconds.

First, change your course and jog backward while you start to swing the jumping string. Make the move within 15 seconds. Full your package by making a hopscotch jump in 15 seconds. Spring rope in position to make the leap, and when you run, alternate between jumping your feet to the sides and then back to the middle, similar to how you'd leap them when jumping jacks. Make the move within 15 seconds. If you're an intermediate exerciser, you can take 30 seconds to perform the steps and 30 seconds to rest between sets. The advanced circuit should be shown for 60 seconds at a time, and 60 seconds of rest should follow.

Aerobic Strength Circuit

This workout improves cardiovascular and heart health, develops energy, and tones major muscle groups.

With each exercise emphasis on the proper shape to avoid injury. Hold the heart rate at an all-time moderate level. In this exercise, you should be able to carry on a brief conversation. This aerobic circuit is conceived to increase the heart rate. For 1 minute, perform the following strength exercises: Then jog or march for 1 minute in place for your active rest. This is one of those circuits. Repeat 2 to 3 times on a circuit. You can rest in between the circuits for up to 5 minutes. Afterward, cool down with some light stretching.

Aerobic Gym Exercises

A great place to get into some aerobic exercise is your nearest gym. They own devices such as treadmills, stationary bikes, and elliptical machines. There may also be a swimming pool for you to play in. If you are not sure how to use any form of exercise equipment, always ask for assistance from a specialist or trainer.

Stationary Bike

A low-impact exercise can help build strength in the legs. Ask a gym trainer to help change the motorcycle, so the seat is the right height. If you are cycling at home, a general rule is to change the seat height of the bike to retain a 5-to 10-degree bend in your knee before it reaches full length. Doing so will reduce compression on the knee joint. Extending the knee entirely when peddling on a stationary bike isn't recommended. Riding a stationary bike is yet another low-impact cardio choice. Stationary bikes are an excellent cardiovascular exercise, they help you develop strength in your legs, and they are easy to use. Most gyms and fitness studios offer classes for cycling, which use stationary bikes. But you can still enjoy a stationary bike workout without having to take a lesson. Having relaxed and warmed up by cycling for 5 to 10 minutes at a quick speed, raise your pace to 15 miles per hour and strive for 20 to 30 minutes of steady cycling. Refrigerate for 5 minutes. Stretch to complete.

Elliptical

Elliptical machines provide a strong cardiovascular exercise that is less taxing on the knees, hips, and back compared to the treadmill or road or trail running. Look on, not down. If you feel shaky, or help you get on and off the machine, use the handlebars. At first, the elliptical machine might seem daunting, but once you get the hang of it, it is easy to use. Keep your body upright after warming up, while using your legs in a pedal movement to push the pump. Look forward the whole time, not your feet down. Keep your shoulders active and your abdominal muscles. Cool down and remove the stretching unit.

Aerobics Class Workouts

If you don't like to exercise alone, a class will provide a friendly and motivating atmosphere. If you're young, ask the professor to show you the appropriate form. If you're a novice, they will help you adjust the exercises, if necessary. Attend group classes for starting 2 to 3 days a week at your nearest fitness center. If you like the workout, you can always go on more often later.

Cardio Kickboxing

Kickboxing is an activity of high impact that creates strength and stamina. It can also reduce stress and make the reflexes stronger. Drink plenty of water over the entire class. If you're feeling dizzy, take a break. Your class can begin by warming up jogging, jumping jacks, or strengthening exercises like pushups. So expect the main exercise to make a series of punches, kicks, and hand attacks. In the end, there may be core exercises or reinforcing them. Term the workout always with a cool down and stretch. Drink plenty of water over the entire class.

Indoor Cycling Class

Cycling lessons indoors build strength and strengthen muscle tone and cardiovascular stamina. Lower the resistance if you get tired or if you feel lightheaded take a break. A cycling class will increase the heart rate, unlike a leisurely bike ride. It may include parts of resistance and climb (incline) for maximum profits from preparation. That will help you build strength and muscle tone. Many classes allow you to "strap" cycling shoes into the saddle. These can normally be leased at your place.

Strength Training

Strength training is a form of physical exercise specializing in using muscle contraction resistance, which builds strength, anaerobic endurance, and skeletal muscle size and bone density. When correctly done, strength training can provide critical functional benefits and improve overall health and well-being, including increased strength and resilience of the bone, muscle, tendon, and ligament, improved joint function, decreased injury risk, increased bone density, increased metabolism, increased activity, and improved cardiac function.

The training uses the technique of gradually increasing muscle force production by small weight changes, and uses a range of exercises and equipment styles to target specific muscle groups. Strength training is predominantly an anaerobic practice, although it has been modified by some advocates by circuit training to provide the advantages of aerobic exercise. Strength training is usually related to lactate development, which is a limiting factor in exercise performance.

Regular endurance exercise leads to skeletal muscle changes that may prevent an increase in lactate levels during strength training.

This is mediated by the activation of PGC-1alpha, which alters the complex composition of the isoenzyme LDH (lactate dehydrogenase) and decreases the activity of the lactate-generating LDHA enzyme while increasing the activity of the lactate-metabolizing LDHB enzyme. Bodybuilding, weightlifting, powerlifting, strongman, highland games, shot put, discus throw, and javelin throw all are sports where strength training is essential. Many other sports, especially tennis, American football, baseball, track and field, rowing, lacrosse, basketball, pole dancing, hockey, professional wrestling, rugby union, rugby league, and soccer, use strength training as part of their training regimen.

Best Strength-Training Moves for Women

Do you want to be strong, safe, happy, and feel ten years younger? It is then time to collect the weights. "Strength training is no longer about being strong or slim." It's as important to your health as mammograms and annual doctor visits, and it can relieve almost all of the physical and emotional problems that women face today. And it becomes even more vital after you reach 50. "That's because women lose up to 5 percent of their lean muscle tissue every decade, beginning in their 30s — and that number increases after 65." The more you build, the quicker the metabolism hums, you get smoother and firmer, and it's easier to lose weight, and hold it off. "It also reduces the risk of diabetes, stroke, and heart disease and makes you less likely to fall or get hurt. Who's on a quest to raise women's weight— the benefits go even deeper.

It's time for women to regain their strength." "Every woman should do a regimen of full-body strength training — such as this one-two day a week. Then, on top of that, you can incorporate other fitness elements such as yoga, dance, biking, or swimming." (Incorporate one of these three new walking exercises that blast fat into your exercise routine.) You can do all of these movements in one workout, or you can split them up if you're short on time.Central to that is continuity. Aim to complete three sets for each move, and choose a weight that makes the final rep of each set difficult. While the gym is a great place for a weight workout, these movements can be made right at home. All you are going to need is a chair, hand weights, and a mat.

1. Squat to Chair

"The best way to maintain and enhance bone density is by movements involving the entire lower body. This move is considered a weight-bearing, complicated, complex movement and is number one for bone health. Furthermore, the pelvis is implicated in most age-related falls and bone fractures. This movement specifically targets and strengthens the pelvis' muscles and bones. "(There are four more strength training movements you can do with a chair.) Stand apart with your feet shoulder-width distance with your toes bent out slightly. Stretch your arms forward and hold them parallel to the floor throughout the movement.

2. Reverse Lunge

This step reinforces the basic movement patterns that control walking, climbing stairs, and the transition from sitting to standing. 'It strengthens your entire lower body and helps keep you as healthy as you wish. 'Stand next to a chair or stable surface to use for support. Keep a 5 to 10-pound dumbbell in your right hand and put your left hand on the chair.

3. Seated Overhead Press

For all women of all ages, one of the toughest movements is pushing upward upwards. "Due to the reduced muscle mass at 50, this vital movement pattern is further handicapped. This activity raises the lean muscle mass around your shoulders, decreasing the risk of spine, shoulder, and lower back injury by pushing a heavy overhead." (Try these three exercises to shape strong shoulders.) Start sitting with your back supported and 5-to 8-pound dumbbells resting on your show. Stand straight, and make sure your elbows are under your wrists. Press up, so the elbows are in front of your chest, not sideways. End with the dumbbells directly above your head, palms forward, maximum extended elbows but not closed. Slowly release after the same sequence of movement, and finish at the starting position. That is a replay. Target 10-12 reps.

4. Standing Calf Raise

One of the biggest concerns, when we age, is the risk of falling, "Perkins says." This step increases your feet and lower legs ' stability and agility, and the ability to know where your body is in space. This sense is called proprioception. "Hold a 10-15 pound dumbbell in your right hand and put your left hand on a chair or stable equilibrium surface. Move your weight to your left foot and raise your right foot off the floor. Stand with a long, straight spine and allow the dumbbell to hang at your side.

5. Bent-over Row

"We are constantly fighting a battle because of gravitational pull to keep our body upright and in good alignment. This step improves all the muscles in your back, increasing both the bone density of the spine and the proper alignment of the spinal column. It also helps combat the deterioration in the bone that happens over 50 and holds your body upright." Standing behind a chair using 8-to 15-pound dumbbells.

Place your feet under your knees and fold forward to allow your head to rest on the chair or surface comfortably. Keep your knees bent slightly and relax your back. Start directly under your shoulders with your palms facing one another. Bend your elbows and pull the dumbbells in your direction until your palms are touching your ribs. At the top, bring the blades of the shoulder together. Pause for two seconds, then release gradually back to starting position. That's one repetition. Look for reps 12 to 15.

6. Superman

"This move is one of the number one encouragement exercises physical therapists are using for back safety. "It strengthens your' posterior chain ' muscles, which guide almost every move you make, including your heart, glutes, back, and shoulder muscles all at once while helping to open your hips and shoulders." Stretch your core muscles, and balance your pelvis and shoulders. Turn the weight to the left knee and right hand. Extend your right leg behind you in one turn, and your left arm outside in front of you. Extend both to the limit and stay for 2 seconds. Return both to starting position gradually. That is a replay. Switch sides immediately and do the same with the left leg and right arm. Continue to switch sides for 20 reps to complete.

7. Chest Fly

"The muscles in the chest (pectorals) are especially weak and underdeveloped for all women. "You add a substantial percentage of lean mass to your overall health by raising the mass in this muscle group. This step will provide a little more lift to your chest. "Place 5-to 8-pound dumbbells in front of each other directly over your arms.

To balance your heart, move your shoulders away from your ears and down into your thighs.

Open your arms with a very slight bend at the elbows until the upper arms touch the floor. Do not completely release the tension in your shoulders, or allow your wrists to touch the floor. Muscle the chest muscles to get the dumbbells back to their starting position. That is a replay. Look for 12 to 15 reps to complete.

8. Dumbbell Pullover

"This step enhances the ability to more comfortably and quickly pull heavy objects. "Moreover, almost all of my 50 + women first talk about the soft tissue on the back of their upper arms. This step directly targets the triceps muscles to add more muscle and strengthening to that region." Place a 10-to 15-pound dumbbell at one end, so that when you stretch your arms upward, the other end is on the floor. Start engaging with your heart and pull down your shoulders from your ears to your hips. Pick the dumbbell off the floor from there. Drop the dumbbell slowly back to the floor, making the same arc. That is a replay. Before lowering the dumbbell fully to the floor, lift it again immediately and complete 12 to 15 repetitions.

9. Biceps Hammer Curl

"From a volume perspective, the muscles of your upper arms are very weak. These muscles are atrophied because of the muscle loss that has occurred since your 30s (sarcopenia). "It's critical to keep your biceps muscles strong so you can carry objects safely and easily. It'll also make your arms look great." (Test this at-home workout for more moves for sculpted arms.) Stand with your feet under your hips and hold 8-to 10-pound dumbbells on your sides with your palms facing inwards.

Stand with a strong, long spine. Bend your elbows and put the dumbbells up to your shoulders, holding each other's palms face up. Bring the dumbbells to the front of the shoulders before they touch.

Have a 2-second pause here and contract the muscles in your upper arms. Lower back to start position slowly. That is a replay. Aim to fill in 10 to 15 reps.

10. Basic Abs

"There is a tendency for women over 50 to grow a distended belly. This action is good for pulling the abdominal muscles inwards towards your spine, making the abdominal muscles stronger and tighter." Place your hands with your upper body relaxed on your thighs. Turn your head slowly into your chest on an exhale and lift it until your shoulders rise off the floor. Your palms float up to your knees. Keep lifting until your shoulders are fully off the table, or your knees touch your fingertips. Stop for 2 seconds at the rim, and then slowly lower back to the starting point. That is a replay. Seek 20 to 30 reps.

Stretching is the form of physical exercise in which a specific muscle or tendon (or group of muscles) is intentionally flexed or extended to increase the perceived elasticity of the muscle and to achieve relaxed muscle tone. The effect is a feeling of increased muscle strength, flexibility, and motion speed. Therapeutically, stretching is also used to soothe cramps. Stretching is a normal and instinctive practice in its most basic form; humans and many other species practice it. It can come with yawning.

Stretching often happens spontaneously after awakening from sleep, after long inactivity periods, or after leaving confined spaces and areas.

One of the basic tenets of physical fitness is to increase flexibility by stretching. Athletes prefer to stretch before (for warming up) and after exercise in an attempt to reduce injury risk and improve performance. If done improperly, stretching can be dangerous.

There are many stretching methods in general, but some strategies may be ineffective or harmful depending on which muscle group is stretched, even to the point of causing hypermobility, weakness, or permanent damage to the tendons, ligaments, and muscle fiber. Therefore, the physiological nature of the stretching and hypotheses about the impact of different techniques are subject to heavy study.

"The older we get, the more likely we are to be tight, and our muscles are pushing into our skeletal structure and throwing us out of whack. Stretching opens up the muscles of the body so that the blood flow increases. "As you stretch, you stretch your muscles around the joint, which helps to increase the range of movement and prevent injury. Stretching can also lower stress, improve mood, and make you feel better in general.

As to how often an older adult can stretch out, "I look at stretching the teeth like flossing. Hopefully, you floss every day, but when you've got food in your teeth too. Stretching is the same, doing it every day will help you feel better, but you can also do it when your muscles feel tight or when your body is feeling heavy. They are quick, productive, and perfect for any adults over 50 who want to stretch out. One thing to note "If there's discomfort, do not keep a static stretch. This is a warning that you are stretching too far and should be going backward. Stretching can be difficult, but it should feel like healthy stress as well.

Arm opener

Stretches your Back, Chest, and Shoulders

Sit apart and flat on the floor with your feet comfortably apart. Take your hands and interlace them with knuckles down below your tailbone. Looking straight ahead and with relaxed muscles, push your arms softly up and away from your tailbone as far as possible. Go to your chest where you feel a nice stretch and take five deep breaths.

Chin Drop

Stretches your neck and shoulders

With your elbows meeting in front of you, and your palms facing you with the sides of your pinkies touching. Use the weight of your arms and place your hands on top of your head; gently lower your chin to where you have a nice stretch in your neck and shoulders. Take five deep breaths in your upper back and release any unnecessary tension into the tightest areas.

Hippie Stretch

Balances your knees, stretches the hamstrings and lower back of your legs,

Place your feet on the ground together and flat. Bend your hips slowly forward and move your hands down your legs, as low as it feels comfortable. So alternate bending one knee and holding the other leg straight (but keeping your feet flat) and lowering your head, releasing all tension. Stretch out for 15 seconds on each side. When one side is tighter, remain there longer to maintain the balance of the muscle.

Hula Hoop Stretch

Warm-up and relax your shoulders, increase mobility, stand together with your feet and hands on your waist. Circle the hips in clockwise five times, and then in counter-clockwise five times. Pretend that a rope from the top of your head elongates your back, resists shifting your arms, holds your stomach pulled in, and concentrates on pushing your hips as wide as possible in a circle.

Overhead Triceps Stretch

Stretches your arms,

Stand apart and roll your shoulders down and back with your feet hip-width apart.

Lift your right arm to the ceiling, holding your head off your face. Bend your right elbow and put your right hand with your palm facing your back towards the center of your return. Upon the roof, raise your left hand and put your fingertips on your right arm just above the elbow. Hold a place in the stretch for 15-30 seconds.

Yo-Yo Stretch

Align your spine and strengthen your posture,

Stand apart with the shoulder-width of your feet and slightly pointed toes. Interlace your hands and carry them to the level of your stomach, about six inches in front of your eyes, with palms facing off your body and your elbows on either side. From this position, and while keeping your lower body stable, move your upper body from side to side to where it feels comfortable, lead with your elbows and keep your head in line with your torso. If you are likely to get dizzy, keep your eyes forward. Do them ten times.

90 Lat Stretch

Spread your back,

Stand apart with the hip-width of your feet and your arms on your sides. Brace your abdominal muscles to get your spine healthy. Bring the blades down and back of your head. Keep your shoulders high, and tilting your head slightly. Shift your weight over your heels with a slight bend in your knees and start bending gradually at the hips.

Hold the abdominals braced, and the back flat. Put your hands down on the table.

Keep your arms straight, so there's a line from the shoulders to the hands, through the elbows. Lean back into your shoulders, straighten your legs and lower your body toward the ground, holding your back flat. Keep your chin tucked in your neck to support your backbone to keep your head from falling towards the floor.

Keep your legs directly under your hips, with your hands on the table. Hold a place in the stretch for 15-30 seconds. Repeat twice–4 times.

Quad pull

Stretches your legs and increases flexibility,

Standing side by side with your feet and back. Place your right hand on a wall or table to support it, then brace your right leg and bend your left knee back up until you can catch the ankle with your left hand. Maintain a straight line up to your tailbone from top of your head. Keep your chest high, take five deep breaths, and then switch sides.

Working out When You're Over 50

A body which is 50 or 60 is not the same as a body which is 20 years old. You're not going to be able to do the same things — and you should not. Yet exercise is vital to your freedom as you age and good quality of life. So what does it take you to think about being safe without harming yourself? As you get older, you lose muscle mass, and exercise will help you regain it.

Even at rest, muscles burn more calories than fat, which will counteract the slowing metabolism. Exercise helps to stop, pause, and at times boost serious diseases such as heart disease, high blood pressure, diabetes, stroke, Alzheimer's disease, arthritis, and osteoporosis. It can help keep your brain focused and keep you from getting into a funk.

Young or old, there are different kinds that everyone wants. Cardio or aerobic exercise picks up your heart rate and helps you breathe faster, increasing your stamina and burning calories. Training with strength or weight leaves the muscles ready for action.

Exercises of flexibility help you stay limber so you can have a full range of movement to avoid injury. After age 50 balances training becomes necessary, so you can prevent falls and stay active. Lower-impact exercise is kinder to your knees, with less jumping and punching in it. Many activities provide more than one type of activity, so your workout dollar will get more bangs. Pick things you love to do! Based on the limitations of any medical conditions you have, your doctor or physical therapist can recommend ways to adapt sports and activities, or better alternatives. Lower-impact exercise is kinder to your knees, with less jumping and punching in it. Many exercises provide more than one type of exercise, so your workout dollar will get more bangs. Pick things you love to do! Based on the limitations of any medical conditions you have, your doctor or physical therapist can recommend ways to adapt sports and exercises, or better alternatives.

Walking

Simple and easy! This enhances the endurance, strengthens muscles in the lower body and helps fight against bone disorders such as osteoporosis. Working up into your day is easy. You can go on solo or socialize this. You will get exercise at a moderate pace, and still be able to chat with a friend or group.

Jogging

If you like to sweat a little more while exercising, try to jog to get your heart rate up. As long as you are taking it slow and steady, wearing the right shoes, and taking breaks to walk, your joints should be fine. Soft surfaces, such as a track or grass, can help too. Pay attention to your calves and hips, with extra stretching and reinforcement to reduce your chances of injury.

Dancing

It doesn't matter what kind of class: ballroom, line, square and dance-based aerobics classes such as Zumba and Jazzercise. Dancing increases endurance strengthens muscles, and improves balance. It uses up a lot of calories because it lets you push in every direction. Learning new moves is also genuinely useful for your brain. Plus, there's so much fun you could have, you might not know you're doing exercise.

Golfing

Much of this sport's benefit comes from walking: an average trip is more than 10,000 steps or about 5 miles! Therefore, the swing uses your entire body, and it requires the right balance— and a steady concentration. If you are wearing your clubs or dragging them, that's even more of a workout. But it's worth using a truck, too. Your muscles are still functioning, and you are taking steps along with fresh air and relief from tension.

Cycling

If you have swollen or sore knees, it's especially good because your legs don't have to bear your weight. The action gets the blood moving and develops muscles on your legs and hips both at the front and back. For balance, you use your abs and steer your arms and shoulders. You're reinforcing the bones because there's resistance, too. Bike frames and saddles, especially designed, will make cycling safer and easier for different health problems.

Tennis

Racquet sports, like tennis, squash, and badminton, may be particularly good at keeping you alive for longer and reducing your chance of dying from heart disease.

Playing tennis 2 or 3 times a week is associated with improved agility and reaction times, lower body fat and higher "healthy" HDL cholesterols.

And it's building bones, especially in your arm, low back, and neck. Play doubles for a more relaxed, less intense workout.

Swimming

You will work out in the water for longer than you do on the ground. There's no weight placing stress on your joints (and making them hurt), and the water provides muscle and bone-building resistance. Swimming laps burns calories, which acts like jogging and running with your face, but you are not likely to overheat. The humidity helps people breathe asthma. Water-based exercise helps people with fibromyalgia in their mentality.

Yoga

Holding a series of poses regularly will stretch and strengthen your muscles, along with the tendons and ligaments that hold your bones together. Breathing deliberately also gives it some kind of meditation. Yoga will help to lower the heart rate and blood pressure, and to relieve anxiety and depression. Check out various styles and classes to suit your fitness level and what appeals to you.

Tai Chi

This relaxing movement is sometimes called "moving meditation." You slowly and gently move your body, shifting from one place to the next while breathing deeply. It's not only good for coordination; it can also improve bone and heart health. It may help in relieving arthritis pain and stiffness. It could even help you get better sleep.

How Much?

You should get at least 150 minutes of moderate aerobic exercise a week if you are in good health. It is better to spread it over three days or more, for at least 10 minutes at a time.

Do spend time working the muscles directly in your thighs, hips, back, stomach, chest, shoulders, and arms at least twice a week. The more you work out, the higher the gain you get. And nothing could be better than nothing.

Start Slow

This is particularly important if you haven't exercised for a while or if you undertake a new activity that your body isn't used to doing. Start with 10 minutes and slowly ramp up the workout for how long, how often, or how intensely. Need some motivation? Track your progress on your own, or with an app or online tool like My Go4Life at the National Institutes of Health.

When to Call Your Doctor

Chest pain, breathing problems, dizziness, problems with balance, and nausea may be warning signs when you are exercising. Instead, let your doctor know earlier. Your body won't recuperate as quickly as it used to. You may have overdone it if the muscles or joints hurt the next day. Turn it back and see what's going on. If the pain continues, consult with your doctor.

3.2 Best Exercise Routines for Women

Age is merely a number. Verily! Looking young, fit and beautiful isn't about how many years you've lived, but how well you've looked after your body. And it should be enjoyed getting to the big five-oh, not feared. These are some of the best female exercise routines in over 50 years. For several reasons, these exercise routines are for women over 50. First of all, those exercises are perfect for muscle building and maintenance.

Naturally, we begin to lose muscle mass as we get older (loss starts as early as age 30!), so it's essential to be vigilant about maintaining tone. To hit all the major muscle groups, these exercises use a mix of dumbbells, bodyweight movements, and exercise machines. They're not going to turn you into a champion in bodybuilding, but they're going to keep you stable through your 50s and beyond. Second, these exercises are a heart-felt challenge without being too taxing. They are perfect for people who are looking to maintain their heart health. Heart disease is the leading cause of death for women in the USA (yikes!), and eating right and exercising regularly are the two main ways to keep the heart-healthy. Such exercises include running, which is performed 3-4 days a week to help keep your heart health going. For women over 50 such activities, as they cover the whole body in multiple ways. We will get you to use your joints, improve your balance, test your endurance, and more. The best way to keep the body youthful is through daily use of it. Keep on going! When you remain active in your 50's, you'll be better off in your 60's and 70's.

10-Minute Beginner's Yoga Workout for Balance

One mistake women frequently make in their 50s is thinking they'll never be able to complete a workout unless they get their first run through it. This Yoga workout aims to improve your balance and flexibility gradually. At first, you can struggle with the poses! Persevere, and you will love the results.

Fitness is not just about being the strongest or the greatest of appearance. Often, exercise is intended to be practical, increasing your range of motion, improve your health, and keep your body from getting older prematurely. Some aspects of functional fitness that gym-goers frequently lack are balance and flexibility.

To absolute beginners, this yoga exercise is intended for health. It's designed to help poorly balanced men. Focus on keeping your body steady while holding each pose for 60 seconds to get the most out of this workout. At first, it could be challenging, but we guarantee it is not impossible! Practice before you master those moves every day. Once you have it down, you can continue to more intense yoga exercises to increase your balance and versatility. A yoga mat for lying down on the floor. Any soft surface, including rubber gym mats, towels, or even soft carpet, will do as well for this workout. Beginning with your right leg forward, keep each pose while breathing deeply for 60 seconds. Then move forwards with your left leg.

Yoga is gaining popularity among older adults, particularly women over 50. Given the numerous benefits that this conventional type of fitness offers, this phenomenon is by no means surprising. Yoga may be a daunting experience, however, particularly if you are exercising for the first time and are totally out of shape. The good news, however, is that you've decided to practice yoga in a holistic way to strengthen yourself. Take a yoga class created exclusively for people like you to make it easier for you. You'll be able to keep your stress levels at bay by starting a gentle session and begin to become active and fit too.

Move and Move, But With Zero Strain

Running alone isn't enough when it comes to safe aging. You need some form of strength training that keeps your agility touchy. The best way of aging healthily and positively, according to physicians, is to practice yoga. Your body will quickly take it away, and you will enjoy it. Yoga strengthens the body by coaxing it softly to engage in a few gentle turns and twists. Since you do not use any external weights, there are zero risks of injury.

You, Will, Enjoy Better Flexibility

You get steeper and less flexible as you age. You will spread out a little more with Yoga. The improved mobility levels allow you to increase the range of your movements as you age. Keeping the spine pliable is essential to avoid getting ridden from the bed.

You Will Be Able To Tackle Menopausal Issues Better

Heat, insomnia, weight gain, dry skin, irritability, osteoporosis are just a few of the menopause women face. For yoga, you can now keep those uncomfortable menopausal symptoms at bay. Whether its hot flashes or back pain, just do a pose for the Boy. You'll feel the difference straight away.

Your Bones Will Have An Extended Lifespan

Brittle bones that cause osteoporosis and fractures are quite common in 50-plus females. Yoga will help to slow the speed at which you experience bone density loss. These will also smooth out the pains and inflammations felt. Research suggests that women over 50 who had been practicing yoga for at least two years acquired mineral density in the bone.

Your Mind Will Remain Sharp

Yoga helps to improve memory and to avoid different cognitive issues related to age. Doing some mild inversion poses, like Downward Facing Dog or Legs up the Wall, may boost blood circulation, keeping your mind sharp.

While you can practice yoga at home by watching videos, I would encourage you to enter a class that does meet your needs. Make sure that you have access to blocks and other yoga accessories, so you can change the poses and stretch yourself to do a little more.

10 Easy Yoga Poses for Women Above 50

If you are a woman over 50, you can try these yoga poses:

1.   **Tadasana – Mountain Pose**

This is one of the easiest of Tadasana, which works well to correct your posture. Make sure you relax with this pose while you go along. Here's what you can expect from Tadasana: more muscular legs, knees, arms and abs, improved metabolism, better breathing, lower stress rates, and better mobility.

2.   **Uttanasana – Standing Forward Bending Pose**

A gentle pose for inversion, this is widely used to treat both osteoporosis and menopause. A gentle exercise in hamstring and hip stretching, it also eases the stress levels. Some of the benefits that Uttanasana provides include improved blood circulation, improved digestive fire, and gentle back massages to ease back pain.

3.   **Adho Mukha Svanasana – Downward Facing Dog Pose**

I simply love the picture. With its endless advantages, you can do it with the utmost ease. But, if you find it challenging to come with hips pointing to the ceiling on your fours, take the help of a tabletop. It is also useful in preventing the onset of osteoporosis, in addition to combating the menopausal pain. Here are a few of the positive effects of this essential yoga asana practice:

Better blood supply,

Eases menopausal pain,

Eases blood pressure,

4.   **Virabhadrasana I – Warrior I Pose**

Using standing yoga pose to strengthen the legs and hips. Only make sure the bones are front-squared and not side-squared. This will mean stronger hips. A wholesome and energizing holistic pose, it also increases the breathing ability. Find out the advantages you will reap from the training Warrior I pose.

Stronger back, knees, thighs, arms, and shoulders,

Opening the eyes, chest and hips, improved flexibility,

Better balance and concentration,

Better circulation, better breathing,

5.   Paschimottanasana – Seated Forward Bend Pose

This pose, along with helping you fight depression and stress, might help you to sleep better. It also wards off tiredness and prepares you to deal better with menopausal problems. This is what you can expect from Seated Bend Pose forwards:

Stretches your lower back,

Hamstrings and spine calms your mind,

Makes you feel nervous and stressful,

6.   Balasana – Child's Pose

Relax like a kid with your eyes lying on the mat while your hands relax next to your chest. It is a crucial pose advocated to promote a sense of relaxation and calmness. It's also useful in strengthening the digestive system and treating menopausal problems better. Check out what you have to tell Balasana.

Helps alleviate tension in the head, chest, and back

7.   Baddha Konasana – Bound Angle Pose

Take care with Baddha Konasana about your wrists, knees, legs, and again with the utmost care. This pose addresses the parts of your body that are more sensitive to discomfort and stress. It also relieves menopausal symptoms along with strengthening the lower back.

8. Ardha Pavanamuktasana – One-Legged Wind Releasing Pose

Type into whatever you want. Then press Quill It on the right to paraphrase your comments. It's a firm, but gentle stretch offered as well as hips to the middle and lower back.

The region's entire muscles get a good massage and time, easing out the nagging backache. So why should you practice Ardha Pavanamuktasana correctly?

9. Bhujangasana – Cobra Pose

Give your back muscles a good stretch, and use this Cobra Pose to strengthen them. To avoid injuries, make sure you keep your shoulders relaxed and rolling backward. If you need additional support, you can save a block under your hands. Thus you benefit from Bhujangasana:

Ease the stiffness of the back,

Improve the strength,

10. Shavasana – Corpse Pose

Use this quick but powerful yoga pose to wind up your yoga class. It's not just a pose for relaxation, but it allows you to gain knowledge of your body and breathing rhythm. So, Shavasana helps you:

Relaxes the mind,

Minimizes anxiety,

Trains the mind,

6-Minute Arm Toning Workout

This workout with a dumbbell arm will show you all the simple lifting exercises you need to tone your muscles. It is going to target your biceps, triceps, shoulders and your upper back a little bit. Beginners should begin with a single round and work their way up gradually from there. You don't need a super-long workout to tone your arms. Using a demanding weight, you have to make the right movements. You'll be targeting the biceps, elbows, triceps, and part of your upper back in this arm toning exercise.

You're going to build strength and lean muscle. Alternatively, this arm toning exercise will help you lose body fat because a higher muscle percentage stimulates your metabolism! To get the most out of your workout, we consider using a punishing dumbbell. Towards the end of each set, you should feel a burn. But make sure you're able to complete the exercise without losing proper form.

What you'll need: a set of light to medium dumbbells (5-15 lb.), a bench, and a gym timer (free apps are available for download.

What to do: perform every move for 45 seconds with 15 seconds of rest in between. Rest for 60 seconds and repeat to make the workout more challenging.

Before Breakfast Mini Morning Workout

There's more energy in a morning workout than a cup of coffee. Not to mention less expensive ones too! This6-minute workout blends yoga with a few simple bodyweight moves to gently wake you up. It will help you stretch, let your blood flow, and even revive your mind.

There are many benefits of working out in the morning. You tend to have more resources first. We are often exhausted and ready to get it over with when we exercise after work or school. Second, morning workouts help to keep you energized for the rest of the day. Ultimately, it helps kick start the various systems in your body, so you're burning calories all day long. To wake you gently, this6-minute workout blends yoga and basic exercises. We built this to be the ideal pick me up before breakfast. It's not too hard, but it's still going to help loosen your muscles, kick your metabolism, and increasing your heart rate.

What you're going to need: a workout timer (free apps are available for download) and a towel to lay on the floor

What to do: perform 40 seconds per step and 20 seconds rest.

How to Tighten Your Butt with Resistance Bands

Just as heightening a heavier weight allows it more potent by adding resistance to a lower-body workout. If you want a genuinely effective ass workout, add your donkey kicks and leg lifts to the resistance bands. You will see results in no time. Donkey kicks are perfect for the gluteus muscles, but you're minimizing their effectiveness when you're using your body weight only. Like any muscle, adding resistance makes the muscle grow faster, achieving results in just a fraction of the time. This is why we suggest doing exercises such as this resistance bands ass workout if you want a better, perkier, rounder behind. Bands of resistance are perfect tools to keep indoors. They are inexpensive, user-friendly, and easy to store. They can go without taking up space in any cabinet. Especially ideal for runners and cyclists is this workout. This exercise by the resistance band will kick your ass to next week!

What you're going to need: a pair of resistance bands (it's easy to buy an inexpensive collection online), a gym timer, and a towel to lay on the floor.

What to do: execute each move for 40 seconds, and pause in between movements for 20 seconds. Complete all moves, and repeat three times in total.

Lose Weight with the Walk Fast/Slow Plan

The strategy will make running more comfortable for you. It's an excellent step-by-step guide for anyone new to running, or people getting back into it after an accident or extended absence.

For many women, all the exercise they need to stay healthy is walking, jogging, or running. Walking appears to be left on the back burner, with workouts like jogging and running getting all the attention.

Walking may seem like simple exercise to some, but it holds a boatload of health benefits. Moderate walking will trim the waist, help maintain weight, and reduce the risk of diseases such as cardiovascular disease and diabetes. Not to mention, work is praising the act of walking because of its ability to boost the level of mood, metabolism, and cognition. Walking is a perfect option for people new to fitness, who have injuries or who just don't want to jog or run. But to make the most of your walking routine, you'll need to add variety. This Lose Weight blends moderate walking with a quicker, more intensive version with the Walk Fast / Slow Program. Powering your muscles through both walking forms will strengthen your muscles and encourage blood flow across your body, and prepare your system for the next level of fitness and complete transformation. You're going to take a break from walking twice a week, and instead do some cross-training. Cross-training offers opportunities for your muscles to rebuild themselves and potentially prevent injury. Not to mention that switching up your workout prevents boredom on the line! Reflect on a mixture of aerobic exercise and strength training during your cross-training days (Ideal for HIIT, Tabata, and circuit training).

Slow walk— Think of this strategy with a concentrated target as a stroll. Tighten your abs, lengthen your back, widen your chest and keep your chin untucked so that there is no constraint on your airway. Do not expend unnecessary energy; slow walking will keep your muscles relaxed, and your heart rate up. When you walk, your forearms should be slightly parallel to the wall.

Quick walk — quick walking or race-walking requires speedier movement of the arm and the legs without the jogging bounce.

On-the-Mat Six Pack Workout

This is a simple workout mat that you can do anywhere, anywhere. After the first few moves, you will find that your abs burns. The key to getting the results noticeable is to keep your heart engaged throughout the workout. Concentrate on keeping abdominal muscles properly developed and contracting. Don't take a stand! You should work straight from the floor for your six-pack abs. This exercise mat is perfect for insulating your abdominals. This uses a series of motions to reach the oblique, lower abs, and upper abs. Start it with a 45-second board that includes the whole body and helps raise your heart rate.

You can do that workout anytime. We suggest it for days when you don't want to go to the gym, or even around an hour before bed as an evening workout.

What you're going to need: a gym timer (free apps are available for download) and a mat or towel to lay on the floor

What to Do: make every move with 15-second breaks in between for 45 seconds. Complete all workouts have a 30-90 second rest, and repeat.

3 Moves to Toned Inner Thighs

This quick3-move workout is a combination of the training on cardio and lower body strength. While the movements will test your muscles and thus make them grow stronger, jumping and walking will also increase your heart rate. Even while you build muscle, you'll be burning calories. Toned inner thighs in shorts are about more than just looking good. Adding power between your legs consistently will help you balance when doing squats, lunges, and deadlifts. It can also help you improve your attitude while you are running or doing yoga. These three motions into toned inner thighs are perfect for any fitness level.

Focus on maintaining proper form to get the most out of this workout. Having the right shape is what really can help you hit those inner thigh muscles, engage them, test them, and make them stronger.

What you're going to need: a pad or towel to lay on the floor

What to do: Finish the workouts in order. Rest and repeat for 60–90 seconds.

Summer Slim Down Workout for Beginners

No treadmill, it's aerobic. But, if you drive this exercise at a fast pace, you'll burn more calories than you'd fly! Squats, walking lunges, hip twists, toe touches, and planks all activate large groups of muscles, which help you burn tons of calories. Do this work out to burn your calories 2 to 3 days a week. Jumping back onto the exercise bandwagon is never too late. An easy exercise is for beginners or anyone who wants to get back into shape. For Beginners, our Summer Slim down Workout uses five basic moves to target different muscle groups. The exercises are easy enough for people of all ages, yet they are genuinely effective at muscle building and calories burning.

What you're going to need: an optional mat or towel to lie on

What to Do: complete the movements to allocate the number of repetitions. If the workout becomes too easy, rest 30-90 seconds and repeat for 2-4 rounds.

10 Yoga Poses for Faster Weight Loss

This is one of the most intense yoga exercises we do. It uses some more demanding positions that get the muscles activated. It's both a great workout to build strength and to lose body fat. That's right; these ten weight-loss yoga poses will help you achieve your fitness goals faster! Many people don't relate exercise to weight loss, but if you take an advanced class in a yoga studio, you're going to do it.

1.   **The Chair**

The chair is like wearing a squat, so it gets the burning of your quads, hamstrings, and calves. And the chair position is perfect for burning calories because it stimulates such large muscle groups.

2.   **Warrior I**

The longer I present the warrior you keep, the more you challenge your thighs. If you start shaking yourself, this means it works!

3.   **Warrior II**

Warrior II is similar to Warrior I, except that it allows you to expand horizontally, stretching, and elongating various areas. Check it out, and the subtle but essential difference you'll find.

4.   **Warrior III**

Try Warrior III when you're very up for a challenge. It seems convenient, but it isn't. Trying to maintain the balance while maintaining the pose will take all the muscles in the hip, heart, and back. You might notice some severe soreness in your legs the first time you are working on this pose.

5.   **Plank Pose**

Planks will get your back, arms, and shoulders engaged. To maintain a proper posture, your body should be in a straight line without sagging or raised hips.

6.   **Boat Pose**

The boat pose requires strong arms to hold onto yourself, so focus on keeping your legs straight and relaxed to prevent straining.

7.   **Downward Dog**

The downward dog is great for your legs and spine stretching, and it's one of the most common positions.

Attaining and maintaining the right form, however, will also involve different muscles in your body, burning calories and increasing the heart rate.

8.   Upward Dog

Upward dog, or upward dog, is a perfect posture to involve your upper body because all your limbs, shoulders, and back will need to work together. It's a great stretch to your stomach and shoulders as well.

9.   Eagle Pose

The eagle pose targets the calf, while at the same time touching other leg muscles. You must also use your back and stomach to keep your body upright rather than bending forward.

10.   Triangle Pose

The triangle pose is our last weight loss yoga pose. It's a perfect posture that works the entire body, including breasts, knees, calves, and shoulders, aligning, and relaxing.

Yoga is a great way to make your fitness healthier and tackle weight loss. It can help you strengthen the muscles and stretch them long. Looking for various ways to incorporate Yoga? Check out 7 Yoga Poses to Tone and describe your arms for runners and 5 Yoga poses.

30-Minute Upper Body Cardio Workout

The 30-minute routine is a full practice session. If you do this, there is nothing else you need to do for the day, other than a fast warm-up and cool-down. This workout on this list is more advanced than some of the others, so it's perfect for already fit women. Don't let anyone make you feel like once you reach 50, you can't be in fantastic shape. You are setting your boundaries! Such training sessions are great for getting on the right track. I hope you like those rituals just as much as I do!

You shouldn't have to sit at the gym for hours to see results. You can get a full upper body workout with this 30-minute interval routine, which is more effective than an hour of lifting. This cardio routine on the upper body incorporates exercises targeting the biceps and shoulders with heart-pumping aerobic movements that torch calories. You'll have three sets of three moves in each for this workout. The shoulder presses and bicep curls will include a pair of dumbbells. Choose demanding weight. You will feel your muscles starting burning by the end of the time limit. Push yourself to work harder and faster with this aerobic exercise on the upper body, and you'll see results in no time!

What you're going to need: a light-to-medium set of dumbbells (5-10 lb.), a gym timer (free apps available for download), and an optional floor layout pad.

What to do: set your timer for an exercise of 45 seconds and a rest of 15 seconds. Cycle through the moves for a total of 3 rounds for each set, with no break in between rounds. Rest 60-90 seconds and proceed to the next game.

Chapter 4: Healthy Lifestyle Habits for Women

4.1 Healthy Habits for Women

Maintaining a healthy lifestyle isn't easy. It is not something that you just find out and forget. This needs an enormous amount of discipline, adaptability, and endurance, spread over everyday life years and years. As you get older, maintaining your health and fitness standard becomes more difficult. Over time things will change, so be ready to adapt. Such ten habits will give you a baseline, and hopefully, forever keep you fit.

1.   Stick to a Solid Sleeping Schedule

Don't underestimate the importance of having the rest of a good evening. Sleep is when the body recovers — whether from exercise, stress, or entirely something else. Having a decent amount of sleep each night was linked to higher productivity, improved exercise skills, and higher mental activity levels. In short, it's essential to sleep.

2.   Follow a Smooth Morning Routine

The most important part of your day may be the morning — or whenever you wake up. That's why you need to build a habit, hold it, and use it as a springboard to set you off for another victory round. It can be an easy morning routine — duster, eat a healthy breakfast, makes your bed, and you're off. May add in some meditation.

3.   Drop the Sugar

Sugar is associated with all sorts of adverse outcomes. The best bets you can make are kicking the habit now and never look back.

Start drinking your black coffee, your sweetener-free tea, and choose a piece of fruit instead of making an ice cream bowl or a snicker.

4.   Concentrate on your Diet

Many of us struggle to regulate our intake, but focusing on the things we eat is one easy way to do so. News & World Report recommends developing a vegetable-based diet— not strictly vegetarian or vegan, but heavy on the greens— and not so reliant on meats, bread, and fats.

5.   Cook more Often

Ever wonder why keeping to a diet is so difficult when you're dining out or depending on packaged foods to get you through the day? It is because you don't have power over what's going into your meal. The best way to fight this obstacle to healthy eating is to make as many of your meals as possible. Eating more homemade meals raises the chances of a higher-quality diet, according to the journal Public Health Nutrition. You could even lose weight. The only "additives" you make in the recipes are those that you add to yourself.

6.   Find ways to Relieve Stress

You'll need to find a way to decompress or to blow some steam off. Some people like going to the shooting range, or playing basketball pickup or soccer. Weight lifting or running to relieve tension is a great habit to get into. Meditation and yoga are other fantastic, stress-relieving habits to pick up in.

7.   Sit Less, Move More

When your job includes sitting for 90 percent of your working day, without even knowing it, you may be harming your safety.

Too much sitting raises the risk for different diseases, in particular heart disease.

Even if you are exercising every day for 30 minutes, spending the next eight hours or more just sitting at a desk ensures that those 30 minutes of exercise are endless. Ideally, you should get up at least every hour and walk a few hundred steps (it only takes a few minutes!).

8.   Drink more Water

Not drinking enough water can lead to both physical and mental fatigue. Evidence also shows you can help lose weight by drinking more water during the day. Some people still confuse hunger and thirst, and end up eating more than they need, so instead of a glass of water, they reach for food.

9.   Spend Time Outdoors

Going outside is better than you think, for your overall health. Notes from Rodale's Organic Life spending time outdoors will help you improve your focus, alleviate stress and anxiety and increasing your intake of vitamin D. A bit of fresh air can have a significant impact on your attitude even for 15 minutes, and take you away from the stress and noise of the crowded indoors.

10.   Learn to Love Exercise

You'll have to work out, at last. And get to learn to love it. Maybe you're a rider, lifter, swimmer, or hiker. It is necessary, however, to develop a love for physical activity and to make it, in some form or another, a pillar of your life. You'll want to get "addicted" to some sort of physical activity, no matter what that is. All you need to do is encourage yourself to see exercise and the rest of these activities as natural aspects of your day, something you enjoy rather than a chore.

Habits of Fit & Healthy Women

The subconscious choices we make every day can impede the efforts that we make to achieve our wellness goals.

Only minor bad habits and negative thoughts can involuntarily prepare us for failure, even if we work hard to succeed. Below is a list of habits and behaviors I've learned that elite women athletes and healthy women have:

1.   They Eat Breakfast

Fit women know that not only does eating the most important meal of the day stimulate their metabolism, but it also gives them the strength to achieve their daily goals. Skipping away at this meal is simply not an option. They're not chowing on sugar donuts, let me be sure. They eat nutritious breakfasts such as Greek yogurt with berries, spinach eggs, or vegetable-filled green juice.

2.   They Eat Snacks Packed with Protein

Healthy women aren't afraid to eat well. Up to six meals a day, they can and will eat: breakfast, snack, lunch, snack, dinner. They don't limit their diets; they eat when hungry – and make smart dietary choices, such as snacking on almonds or berries.

3.   They make Sleep a Priority

Healthy women know that when they are sleep deprived and cranky, they tend to make bad food and lifestyle choices, such as getting the sugar cookie or salty bag of chips. We make sure we get a decent night's sleep, sufficient time to rejuvenate, alleviate stress on the body, rest sore muscles, and refresh.

4.   They don't Drink their Calories

For the most part, fit, women drink water. They limit their intake of caffeine and opt for water to hydrate using lemon, coconut water, and green tea and freshly squeezed green juices.

5.   They have a Positive Relationship with Food

Healthy women recognize that food is meant for fuel and make decisions based on that mindset.

We also made an effort to work without modifying certain emotional eating attachments. Healthy and healthy women pride themselves on nourishing their bodies in the best possible way.

6.   They Allow Themselves to Eat Treats without Guilt

No mind games— all pure chocolate joy, not judgmental. People who associate shame with chocolate cake consumption are more likely to have less control over their diet, and less likely to keep their weight. Healthy women consider chocolate and other candy snacks as sweets— which they rarely have and which are not entirely off-limits.

7.   They Find Creative ways to be Active

You will find healthy women with big grocery bags taking the stairs, going for a brisk walk and smiling at lunch, or doing bicep curls with. Healthy women convert daily tasks into opportunities for calorie loss and muscle toning.

8.   They Laugh Loud and Often

Laughter soothes discomfort, which can result in weight gain and unhealthy habits. If the body is anxious, it causes glucose release. Daily stress does not necessitate all that extra glucose that induces insulin release. The glucose is then transferred to stored fat by insulin.

9.   They Don't Weigh Themselves

Fit women know when they have a good look and feel. To confirm the impression, they do not need a scale or dress size.

10.   They Don't Compare Themselves to Each Other

People with the same BMI will calculate entirely differently. Healthy women do not equate themselves to others for that reason. We are all worried about how we feel and how involved they are.

11. They know that the Gym is not just to be Interested in Working Out

An outdoor outing with friends, cycling, a brisk walk around the mall, hiking, sports, swimming, and yoga are all perfect ways to increase your heart rate and stay fit.

12. They Believe in Balance

Fit women know extreme diets, excessive workouts, and a rigid schedule are not sustainable. By building for a healthy life in habitual wellness practices, they opt for a sensible lifestyle.

13. Set Goals & Plan Ahead

Healthy women have a week's schedule. They don't beat themselves every single day about sticking to the plan, but they know they won't miss out if they devote themselves to a few days a week at the gym or their favorite class. Even once a week, they take a little extra time to plan their healthy meals.

14. Cook Once, Eat Twice

One of the best routines I've built over time is preparing food in bulk so that the next day I can use the leftovers from dinner in my lunch. I mean, the rubbish is boring, right? Don't worry. For instance, if I make roasted veggies for dinner one night with an egg and avocado, I will use the roasted veggies to make a veggie wrap with hummus and a bit of my favorite cheese for lunch.

15. Don't Compare

The root cause of all evils is to compare you to others. It sparks resentment, envy, straight-forwardness, and frustration that contribute to an unhealthy gal. Next time you want to be the person with the glowing skin or thin legs, note your amazing qualities: indoors and outdoors.

16.   Express Gratitude

Showing or remembering how thankful you are in your life for different things will reduce depression and improve immunity. Sounds wild kind of, right? But the relation between our emotions, moods, and brain chemistry is a complex one that can lead to better well-being if care is taken. Try to write down 3-5 items in a gratitude journal every night or morning, and watch the magic happen.

17.   Regular Physical Activity

No brainer, huh? Get up and get out! Whether it's walking, yoga, cycling, spinning, jumping, kickboxing, biking, or swimming, exercise has tremendous benefits, including endorphin release, weight management, improved sleep, enhanced memory, strength, and self-confidence. Try to relax with your body and do a workout that feels right for you. I love running, but it's not everyone's best exercise. Choose your favorite studio if yoga calls to you, and make it a routine. It's important to be consistent in making it a routine and something you look forward to. And keep yourself on track; find a workout buddy who likes to hold you accountable for the same types of exercise as you do.

18.   Eat Whole, Real Food

Here's the thing, what you put in you get out of here. Your body needs fuel of high quality to work at optimum levels, so try eating food with five or fewer ingredients— the healthier the less! Fruit, vegetables, eggs, nuts, and seeds are perfect examples of safe, whole, genuine food. If you've ever had skin swings, digestive swings, bloating swings, or mood swings, I guarantee this little trick will improve tenfold.

19.   Check Your Labels

Some truth lies on the label of your favorite meal. Check it out before you buy to ensure you know all the main ingredients. Rule of thumb: You don't want to eat it if you can't pronounce it. Apart from being able to pronounce the things that go into your mouth, sugar is added to the primary aspect that you want to look out for in your favorite food. White sugar is processed heavily and should be avoided. Eventually, choose foods that have a shortlist of ingredients. My magic number is five or less.

20.   They Have Fun

Although healthy women like having a plan packed with healthy activities such as making home cooking and going to barre, they like having fun as well. Being safe doesn't have to be another hassle in life, and shouldn't. Life is all about striking a balance that will make you feel good and blend into your life. I don't want to make any assumptions, but I will say that it's not going to give you the best attitude to slave away in the gym seven days a week and just eat raw salads. Note, allowing yourself space for spontaneity and the permission to let loose is okay. The healthiest thing you could do is occasionally avoiding the gym and going for drinks and games with the ladies.

21.   Keep Stress at Bay

Stress manifests itself in extremely negative ways inside our bodies, from weight gain to anxiety and mood swings. Comprehending what stresses you out and how it affects your body is important for your overall health. Recognizing your stress factors will allow you to take action immediately. Find ways to calm your mind and relax or things that help you destress.

22.   Consider what goes on Your Body

If we talk about wellness, we usually think about the food that we consume. What we often fail to realize is that what we put on our skin is important. Most shampoos, lotions, and even products for cleaning contain toxic materials, which may be detrimental to our overall health. Just read your mark, just like with food!

23.   Hydrate

Our bodies are composed primarily of water, so we need to drink a lot of it to preserve our health.

Many of us are dehydrated chronically, despite having access to plenty of clean water. For proper circulation, digestion, healthy skin, water is essential, and it also transports other nutrients to the rest of your body. And how much do you have to be drinking? Cut your body weight in half in pounds, and this is how many ounces you can drink. If you're burning your H20 and sweating it out, you'll want to drink more. Try getting an additional eight once.

24.   Self-Care

Many of us are continually looking out for the well-being of others and unable to consider taking care of ourselves. They justify ignoring our own needs by claiming that it is selfish or feeling, "I don't need that," but there's a reason airlines are asking you to put your oxygen mask on first. If you don't have the energy to take care of yourself, there's nothing left for you to devote to others and to give your best self. So go for it: get a massage, a pedicure or take a nice salt bath with the Epsom.

25.   Use the Power of your Mind

You're every girl, so you're sure to have a lot going on in your life–social experience in the rockin, a great career, a gym membership, and a fantastic side hustle or hobby. Moving from task to task with no thought can be easy; being conscious is a vital and powerful resource for your overall health.

It helps you to concentrate and be present, which means you have better workouts, do not over-eat, and respond to stressful situations calmly and coolly. Everyone has different ways to manipulate their consciousness, but my favorite way is fast and easy to do from anywhere: concentrate on your breath. Give it a shot, next time you feel tired, or even as soon as you wake up, close your eyes, take ten deep, slow inhalations and exhales, while concentrating on your body's sensations.

26.   Try Something New

When we do things we know and are good at, many of us feel comfortable and secure. At the same time, trying new things and getting beyond our comfort zone can be both terrifying and exciting. Yet accepting all of the emotions that come with it can bring tremendous benefits related to health. You will experience personal growth and exploration and an ideal mental state when you challenge yourself. For everyone, this might mean something different. For some, it might be going to a new workout class or a film alone; for others, it's getting educated about something you're passionate about; and for some, it's jumping over a beautiful landscape from an airplane. Whatever it means to try something new for you, give it a shot and move your limits beyond, the discomfort will open up new emotions and possibilities where you may also discover a part of yourself you never knew existed.

4.2 Eat Healthy, Stay Fit and Live Well Over 50

You already know saturated fats are harmful to your arteries and heart health. But they can also damage your memory and your concentration. So stop on the red meat, butter, and other things like that. Instead, incorporate more fatty fish and plant fats, such as flaxseed and nuts. Such healthy fats could have additional benefits for your heart and brain.

If your kids are moving out and your house is feeling lonely, consider adopting a cat. Those with cats and dogs tend to have lower cholesterol and lower heart disease risk. They need fewer visits from doctors, too. We don't know precisely why pets seem to be helpful. But at least having a dog that requires walks is a great way to build up in everyday exercise. Growing older doesn't mean doing away with your morning run. People used to believe running was going to wreck their knees. Yet new research suggests it could strengthen them. And it doesn't seem to increase the arthritis risk. That said, running can be too difficult if you have arthritis or damaged joints. Yet you can still enjoy exercise. Low-impact activities such as walking or biking can help reinforce muscles, support joints, and reduce pain. As you get older, your sex life changes— and real benefits will come in. You have had sex for quite a while. You are in it so much better than when you were 22. Getting older can relieve you of hang-ups and restrictions, particularly if your children have moved out, and you have the house back to yourself.

Surprise yourselves. Instead of sticking to the familiar and comfortable stuff, try something different. Go into areas that are out of the ordinary. Make friends. Learn a language or musical instrument. New experiences will build new brain pathways and keep your mind safe as you age. We will extend the possibilities to find fun and joy, too. Does your blood pressure surpass what it used to be? That is not unusual. As we get older, it tends to rise. Cut on salt in your diet, as sodium will push your readings up. Bread and rolls can get a lot of salt, too. Want a natural cure? Eat a banana — potassium can decrease the sodium effect in your diet and may reduce your blood pressure.

Do you want to keep your mind sharp as you grow older? Get pushed.

Daily middle age exercise will lower the chances of having memory and thought problems when you're nearly half more past. Use increases blood flow to your brain and helps to grow new cells there. Only 30 minutes ' walk, bike, or even five days a week gardening will make a difference. Try a wearable fitness tracker, log the food you eat onto a smartphone app or use devices like a home blood pressure monitor to get a complete picture of your health. You will discover new ways to improve your health and to assess your success. So in your 30s and 40s, you weren't getting the healthiest habits. Perhaps you ate too much and were doing too little. That's all right. The goal now is to do better. Changing your lifestyle in your 60s and beyond— more exercise and healthier eating— still can make a big difference. You will reduce your risk of heart issues, cancer, and bone fractures. It just isn't too late. Today, you can be happier and fitter than when you were 30. As you get older, you slow down your metabolism, and you need fewer calories. So do count the ones you get—select foods filled with the requisite nutrients. Eat dark greens of leafy vegetables and colorful fruits. Raise low-fat milk to get bone calcium. Fortified foods— including vitamin B12 cereals and vitamin D milk— can also be of benefit. Delete from sugary drinks and candy on empty calories.

One of the good methods to prevent a fall is to have the right balance— and potentially severe injuries. Consider those workouts part of your day. Stand on one foot or walk heel-to-toe— as though you walked on a platform. Another beneficial choice is the gentle, dance-like movements of Tai chi. older people who stick six months with tai chi can cut their risk of falling in half. Aerobic exercise is essential, but don't forget your muscle-building too. One research in seniors on regular strength training showed that it induced genetic changes in cells. The result: The muscles of older folks in their 20s became more similar to those of men.

Spend some more time with family or friends. It can help you keep a keen mind. Social people have better insight and are far less likely to have problems with memory as they age. And consider doing volunteering. It's linked to lower heart disease risk and longer life. Do not wait until you start withdrawal. The earlier you start, the less likely you will have later on health problems. Does your skin want to question those years? Every day, using sunscreen: it prevents wrinkles. And it's not too late— even people who have not begun to use it until the middle ages are still getting a boost. Choose a product that has a 30 or higher SPF. These days you might need somewhat less sleep than you used to. It is natural. But if you get less than seven hours a night or feel stressed out in the daytime, something is wrong. Insomnia is not a common aspect of aging. Do more exercise, drink less alcohol, and talk to your doctor about your medicine. If you have an underlying problem, such as depression or anxiety, seek treatment; it can help you get back to sleep. Here is some good news: the older people get, the more content they get and the happier they are. People reported being happier in their 80s than individuals in their 70s and looking forward to the future, then. It might be a time of great bliss.

For many women, turning 50 is the start of a life transition. For some, it's when our little ones are not little any more. It could be financial pressure for others or other adult issues. It's a time for females as our bodies change. For example, 51 is the average age of menopause, a natural biological phase defined by the menstrual cycle ending. Shedding weight becomes more difficult for men after they reach 50. With that said, we've got many younger 50-year-olds running around than we've ever seen in the past. What can we attribute this overall improved safety to? First, I think it's because the smoking rates have fallen. Therefore, people are more aware of their diet and exercise these days.

Here are several tips – let's call them ten healthy habits – for keeping your body in good shape after you reach 50:

- **Catch your Z's**

Make sure that you get a good practice of sleep, every day. As we age, our sleep pattern starts to diminish to a period of 23 hours a day. You will, of course, begin to wake up earlier, without an alarm clock. You may not be in a position to stay up as late as you used to, so go with the flow. Hit the sack every day at the same time, and go for as much rest as possible.

- **Exercise**

Our exercise needs to start shifting in the '50s. We need to be aware of the effects of workouts that carry weight on the joints. So, do more muscle cross-training and stretching, which can help to reduce injuries and back pain.

- **Relax**

Learn techniques for relaxation and stress management, and prepare for activities that might be difficult to come. These days, not only do much 50-year-olds care for their older children, but they may also need to care for older parents. That can be pretty stressful. Yoga, meditation, or only a calming walk every day can become your new favorite routine.

- **Brush your Teeth**

The young ones may have been advised to practice good dental health. That's becoming more and more relevant for those over 50, too. Coronary disease is related to gum disease and poor dental hygiene. Getting used to raising your oral health now can reduce that risk in the future.

- **Plan for your Future**

Most people are carrying out a financial review at this stage of their lives. We should all review our health care advance directives, including a living will, a permanent attorney's power, and do - not resuscitate orders, if that is what you might choose. Through regulation, if you don't have long-lasting health care control, the responsibility lies with your spouse, eldest children, or parents. Talk to your older kids about that. Fill out the paperwork so that you name those around you who are confident and responsible for making those choices.

- **Quit Smoking for Good**

Quit all types of tobacco. It could be your last chance to mitigate your heart attack and stroke risks. Stroke risk normalizes after years of leaving in fiver. After ten years, the risk of lung cancer decreases to half that of a smoker.

- **Manage your Weight**

This tip is perhaps the hardest to execute. That's because, because of that metabolism, it's harder to lose weight as you age. Now, set targets for reducing your abdominal fat and central fat. It needs a diet and exercise combination, so eat some vegetables.

- **Protect your Skin**

Daily sun protection is bigger than when you were a young adult. Staying out of the way of harm can lower your risk of non-melanoma skin cancer, which will increase over the next 15-20 years.

- **Get Preventive Screenings**

Know which new preventive tests to apply to your diet, including screening for colon cancer and the Shingrix shingles vaccine. That needs to begin at age 50. Users will often ask at certain ages what scans they should be having. The doctor's go-to preventive care in the United States. Task Force on Preventive Care because it is the most extensive.

- **Moderate your Alcohol Intake**

Limit alcohol consumption to no more than seven women's drinks a week and no more than 14 men's drinks a week.

Dear reader, if you liked this book, let others know your experience, leave your feedback. It will be a pleasure for me to grow and improve thanks to your contribution! Thank you.

https://www.amazon.com/review/create-review/ ref=cm_cr_othr_d_wr_but_top?ie=UTF8&channel=glance-detail&asin=B086BNV752

Conclusion

Health and fitness is a very essential aspect of life which includes physically and mentally fit body. An individual can improve his or her health and fitness with the aid of a healthy diet and regular exercise. While weight loss may seem more challenging with age, many evidence-based approaches may help you achieve and maintain healthy body weight after turning 50. Cutting out added sugars, integrating strength training into your workouts, consuming more protein, cooking meals at home, and adopting a whole-food diet are just some of the ways you can boost your overall health and wellbeing. Good health means a person is healthy physically and mentally, and fitness refers to the person's ability to meet environmental demands. The person who has good health and fitness will thoroughly enjoy his / her life. An individual can achieve good health and fitness by having daily exercise and a proper diet. Not only does it make the person happier, but it also frees him/her from tension and worries. It's important to understand that we can perform our duties properly in life only by paying attention to our body's health and fitness levels.

Therefore we may not be able to attain our goals in life. Being an athlete isn't needed to have a good body. Each person in the world needs a healthy, fit body to stay away from illness and have a long, healthy life. We also need to note how important we are for our families and society. The family members also get trouble if we suffer from diseases. It also impacts their wellness and health. The subconscious choices we make every day can impede the efforts that we make to achieve our wellness goals. Only minor bad habits and negative thoughts can involuntarily prepare us for failure, even if we work hard to succeed. I've spent a lot of time with other happy, fit women as a lifelong athlete.

Our exercise needs to start shifting in the '50s. They need to be aware of the effects of workouts that carry weight on the joints. So, do more muscle cross-training and stretching, which can help to reduce injuries and back pain.

Healthy women recognize that food is meant for fuel and make decisions based on that mindset. They also made an effort to work without altering specific emotional eating attachments. Healthy and healthy women pride themselves on nourishing their bodies in the best possible way. For the most part, fit women drink water. They restrict their consumption of caffeine and opt for water to hydrate using lemon, coconut water, green tea, and freshly squeezed green juices. Healthy women know that when they are sleep deprived and cranky, they tend to make bad food and lifestyle choices, such as getting the sugar cookie or salty bag of chips. We make sure we get a decent night's sleep, sufficient time to rejuvenate, alleviate stress on the body, rest sore muscles, and refresh.

For many women, turning 50 is the start of a life transition. For some, it's when our little ones are not little any more. It could be financial pressure for others or other adult worries. It's a time for females when our bodies change. For example, 51 is the average age of menopause, a natural biological phase defined by the menstrual cycle ending. Shedding weight becomes more difficult for women after they reach 50. With that said, we've got far younger 50-year-olds running around than we've ever seen in the past. What can we attribute this overall improved safety to? Second, I think it's because the smoking rates have fallen.

Furthermore, people, these days are more aware of diet and exercise. A body which is 50 or 60 is not the same as a body which is 20 years old. Yet exercise is vital to your freedom as you age and good quality of life.

So what does it take you to think about being safe without harming yourself? As you get older, you lose muscle mass, and exercise will help you regain it. Exercise helps to stop, pause, and at times boost serious diseases such as heart disease, diabetes, stroke, Alzheimer's disease, arthritis, and osteoporosis. It can help keep your brain focused and keep you from getting into a funk. Young or old, there are different kinds that everyone wants. Cardio or aerobic exercise picks up your heart rate and helps you breathe faster, increasing your stamina and burning calories. Training with strength or weight leaves the muscles ready for action. Exercises of flexibility help you stay limber so you can have a full range of movement to avoid injury. After age 50 balances training becomes necessary, so you can prevent falls and stay active.

Lower-impact exercise is kinder to your knees, with less jumping and punching in it. Many exercises provide more than one type of use, so your workout dollar will get more bangs. Pick things you love to do! Depending on the limitations you have of any medical conditions, your doctor or physical therapist can recommend ways to adapt sports and exercises, or better alternatives. Yoga is gaining popularity among older adults, particularly women over 50. Given the numerous benefits that this conventional type of fitness offers, this phenomenon is by no means surprising. Yoga may be a daunting experience, however, particularly if you are exercising for the first time and are totally out of shape. The good news, however, is that you've decided to practice yoga in a holistic way to strengthen yourself. Take a yoga class created exclusively for people like you to make it easier for you. You should be able to control the stress levels at bay by starting a gentle session and begin to become active and fit too.

References

- Tremblay MS, e. Physiological and health implications of a sedentary lifestyle. - PubMed - NCBI. Retrieved from **https://www.ncbi.nlm.nih.gov/pubmed/21164543**
- G, S. Evidence based exercise - clinical benefits of high intensity interval training. - PubMed - NCBI. Retrieved from **https://www.ncbi.nlm.nih.gov/pubmed/23210120**
- High-Intensity Interval Training: An Alternative for Older Adults - Michael Whitehurst, 2012. Retrieved from **https://journals.sagepub.com/doi/10.1177/1559827612450262**
- The 20 Best Ways to Lose Weight After 50. Retrieved from **https://www.healthline.com/nutrition/how-to-lose-weight-after-50**
- These Doctor-Approved Diets Help Women Over 50 Fulfill All Their Health Needs. Retrieved from **https://www.womansday.com/health-fitness/nutrition/a30550619/best-diets-for-women-over-50/**
- 10 Best Weight Loss Tips For Women Over 50. Retrieved from **https://skinnyms.com/best-weight-loss-tips-for-women-over-50/**
- Weiler, L. The Metabolism-Boosting Tips Everyone Over 50 Needs to Know. Retrieved from **https://www.cheatsheet.com/health-fitness/the-metabolism-boosting-tips-everyone-over-50-needs-to-know.html/**
- Cold, F., Health, E., Disease, H., Disease, L., Management, P., & Conditions, S. et al. Get-Fit Tips for Women Over 50. Retrieved from **https://www.webmd.com/women/guide/women-over-50-fitness-tips**

- 10 Best Strength-Training Moves For Women Over 50. Retrieved from https://www.prevention.com/fitness/a20479225/best-strength-training-exercises-for-women-over-50/ (These are described in Chapter 3, under 3.1)

- Best Exercise Routines for Women Over 50. Retrieved from https://skinnyms.com/best-exercise-routines-for-women-over-50-10/ (These are described in Chapter 3, under 3.2)

- The 5 Crucial Diet Changes Women Over 50 Must Make. Retrieved from https://www.theactivetimes.com/healthy-living/nutrition/5-crucial-diet-changes-women-over-50-must-make

- The 10 Best New Exercises for Women. Retrieved from http://www.oprah.com/health/the-10-best-new-exercises-for-women/all

- Wasser, L. The Benefits of Exercise Over 50 - RedTea News. Retrieved from https://redtea.com/news/the-benefits-of-exercise-over-50/

- 5 Tips for Women to Stay Fit After 50. Retrieved from https://health.clevelandclinic.org/5-tips-to-stay-fit-after-50-2/

- Physical fitness. Retrieved from https://en.wikipedia.org/wiki/Physical_training